The Etiology
and Prevention
of Drug Abuse
Among Minority Youth

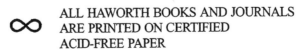

The Etiology and Prevention of Drug Abuse Among Minority Youth

Gilbert J. Botvin, PhD
Steven Schinke, PhD
Editors

The Haworth Press, Inc.
New York • London

The Etiology and Prevention of Drug Abuse Among Minority Youth has also been published as *Journal of Child & Adolescent Substance Abuse*, Volume 6, Number 1 1997.

The development, preparation, and publication of this work has been undertaken with great care. However, the publisher, employees, editors, and agents of The Haworth Press and all imprints of The Haworth Press, Inc., including The Haworth Medical Press and Pharmaceutical Products Press, are not responsible for any errors contained herein or for consequences that may ensue from use of materials or information contained in this work. Opinions expressed by the author(s) are not necessarily those of The Haworth Press, Inc.

Cover design by Thomas J. Mayshock, Jr.

The Haworth Press, Inc., 10 Alice Street, Binghamton, NY 13904-1580 USA

Library of Congress Cataloging-in-Publication Data

The etiology and prevention of drug abuse among minority youth / Gilbert J. Botvin, Steven Schinke, editors.
     p. cm.
     "Has also been published as Journal of child & adolescent substance abuse, volume 6, no. 1, 1997"–Verso CIP t.p.
     Includes bibliographical references and index.
     ISBN 0-7890-0330-9 (alk. paper)
     1. Minority youth–Drug use–United States. 2. Youth–Drug use–United States. 3. Drug abuse–United States. 4. Minority youth–Drug use–United States–Prevention. 5. Youth–Drug use–United States–Prevention. 6. Drug abuse–United States–Prevention. I. Botvin, Gilbert J. II. Schinke, Steven Paul.
HV5824.Y68E848 1997
362.29′0835′0973–dc21

                                  97-16110
                                   CIP

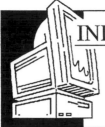

INDEXING & ABSTRACTING

Contributions to this publication are selectively indexed or abstracted in print, electronic, online, or CD-ROM version(s) of the reference tools and information services listed below. This list is current as of the copyright date of this publication. See the end of this section for additional notes.

- *Academic Abstracts/CD-ROM*, EBSCO Publishing Editorial Department, P.O. Box 590, Ipswich, MA 01938-0590

- *ALCONLINE Database*, Swedish Council for Information on Alcohol and Other Drugs, Box 27302, S-102 54 Stockholm, Sweden

- *Biology Digest*, Plexus Publishing Company, 143 Old Marlton Pike, Medford, NJ 08055

- *Brown University Digest of Addiction Theory and Application, The (DATA Newsletter)*, Project Cork Institute, Dartmouth Medical School, 14 South Main Street, Suite 2F, Hanover, NH 03755-2015

- *Cambridge Scientific Abstracts, Health & Safety Science Abstracts,* Environmental Routenet (accessed via INTERNET), 7200 Wisconsin Avenue #601, Bethesda, MD 20814

- *Child Development Abstracts & Bibliography*, University of Kansas, 2 Bailey Hall, Lawrence, KS 66045

- *CINAHL (Cumulative Index to Nursing & Allied Health Literature), in print, also on CD-ROM from CD PLUS, EBSCO, and SilverPlatter, and online from CDP Online (formerly BRS), Data-Star, and PaperChase. (Support materials include Subject Heading List, Database Search Guide, and instructional video.)*, CINAHL Information Systems, P.O. Box 871/1509 Wilson Terrace, Glendale, CA 91209-0871

- *CNPIEC Reference Guide: Chinese National Directory of Foreign Periodicals*, P.O. Box 88, Beijing, People's Republic of China

- *Criminal Justice Abstracts*, Willow Tree Press, 15 Washington Street, 4th Floor, Newark, NJ 07102

- *Current Contents . . . . see: Institute for Scientific Information*

- *Educational Administration Abstracts (EAA)*, Sage Publications, Inc., 2455 Teller Road, Newbury Park, CA 91320

(continued)

- *ERIC Clearinghouse on Counseling and Student Services (ERIC/CASS)*, University of North Carolina-Greensboro, 101 Park Building, Greensboro, NC 27412-5001

- *Exceptional Child Education Resources (ECER), (CD/ROM from SilverPlatter)*, The Council for Exceptional Children, 1920 Association Drive, Reston, VA 20191

- *Family Life Educator "Abstracts Section,"* ETR Associates, P.O. Box 1830, Santa Cruz, CA 95061-1830

- *Family Studies Database (online and CD/ROM)*, National Information Services Corporation, 306 East Baltimore Pike, 2nd Floor, Media, PA 19063

- *Health Source: Indexing & Abstracting of 160 selected health related journals, updated monthly*, EBSCO Publishing, 83 Pine Street, Peabody, MA 01960

- *Health Source Plus: expanded version of "Health Source" to be released shortly*, EBSCO Publishing, 83 Pine Street, Peabody, MA 01960

- *Index to Periodical Articles Related to Law*, University of Texas, 727 East 26th Street, Austin, TX 78705

- *Institute for Scientific Information*, 3501 Market Street, Philadelphia, Pennsylvania 19104-3302 (USA). Coverage in:
  a) Social Science Citation Index (SSCI): print, online, CD-ROM
  b) Research Alert (current awareness service)
  c) Social SciSearch (magnetic tape)
  d) Current Contents/Social & Behavioral Sciences (weekly current awareness service)

- *International Bulletin of Bibliography on Education*, Proyecto B.I.B.E./Apartado 52, San Lorenzo del Escorial, Madrid, Spain

- *INTERNET ACCESS (& additional networks) Bulletin Board for Libraries ("BUBL"), coverage of information resources on INTERNET, JANET, and other networks.*
  - JANET X.29: UK.AC.BATH.BUBL or 00006012101300
  - TELNET: BUBL.BATH.AC.UK or 138.38.32.45 login 'bubl'
  - Gopher: BUBL.BATH.AC.UK (138.32.32.45). Port 7070
  - World Wide Web: http: // www.bubl.bath.ac.uk./BUBL/ home.html
  - NISSWAIS: telnetniss.ac.uk (for the NISS gateway)
  The Andersonian Library, Curran Building, 101 St. James Road, Glasgow G4 0NS, Scotland

(continued)

- *Medication Use STudies (MUST) DATABASE*, The University of Mississippi, School of Pharmacy, University, MS 38677
- *Mental Health Abstracts (online through DIALOG)*, IFI/Plenum Data Company, 3202 Kirkwood Highway, Wilmington, DE 19808
- *National Criminal Justice Reference Service*, National Institute of Justice/NCJRS, Mail Stop 2L/1600 Research Boulevard, Rockville, MD 20850
- *NIAAA Alcohol and Alcohol Problems Science Database (ETOH)*, National Institute on Alcohol Abuse and Alcoholism, 1400 Eye Street NW, Suite 600, Washington, DC 20005
- *Psychological Abstracts (PsycINFO)*, American Psychological Association, P.O. Box 91600, Washington, DC 20090-1600
- *Referativnyi Zhurnal (Abstracts Journal of the Institute of Scientific Information of the Republic of Russia)*, The Institute of Scientific Information, Baltijskaja ul., 14, Moscow A-219, Republic of Russia
- *Sage Family Studies Abstracts (SFSA)*, Sage Publications, Inc., 2455 Teller Road, Newbury Park, CA 91320
- *Sage Urban Studies Abstracts (SUSA)*, Sage Publications, Inc., 2455 Teller Road, Newbury Park, CA 91320
- *Social Planning/Policy & Development Abstracts (SOPODA)*, Sociological Abstracts, Inc., P.O. Box 22206, San Diego, CA 92192-0206
- *Social Science Citation Index . . . . see: Institute for Scientific Information*
- *Social Work Abstracts*, National Association of Social Workers, 750 First Street NW, 8th Floor, Washington, DC 20002
- *Sociological Abstracts (SA)*, Sociological Abstracts, Inc., P.O. Box 22206, San Diego, CA 92192-0206
- *Special Educational Needs Abstracts*, Carfax Information Systems, P.O. Box 25, Abingdon, Oxfordshire OX14 3UE, United Kingdom
- *Studies on Women Abstracts*, Carfax Publishing Company, P.O. Box 25, Abingdon, Oxfordshire OX14 3UE, United Kingdom
- *Violence and Abuse Abstracts: A Review of Current Literature on Interpersonal Violence (VAA)*, Sage Publications, Inc., 2455 Teller Road, Newbury Park, CA 91320

(continued)

SPECIAL BIBLIOGRAPHIC NOTES

related to special journal issues (separates)
and indexing/abstracting

☐ indexing/abstracting services in this list will also cover material in any "separate" that is co-published simultaneously with Haworth's special thematic journal issue or DocuSerial. Indexing/abstracting usually covers material at the article/chapter level.

☐ monographic co-editions are intended for either non-subscribers or libraries which intend to purchase a second copy for their circulating collections.

☐ monographic co-editions are reported to all jobbers/wholesalers/approval plans. The source journal is listed as the "series" to assist the prevention of duplicate purchasing in the same manner utilized for books-in-series.

☐ to facilitate user/access services all indexing/abstracting services are encouraged to utilize the co-indexing entry note indicated at the bottom of the first page of each article/chapter/contribution.

☐ this is intended to assist a library user of any reference tool (whether print, electronic, online, or CD-ROM) to locate the monographic version if the library has purchased this version but not a subscription to the source journal.

☐ individual articles/chapters in any Haworth publication are also available through the Haworth Document Delivery Services (HDDS).

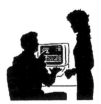

The Etiology and Prevention of Drug Abuse Among Minority Youth

CONTENTS

ABOUT THE EDITORS

Gilbert J. Botvin, PhD, is Professor of Public Health and Psychiatry and Director of the Institute for Prevention Research at Cornell University Medical College in New York, New York. An international leader in research on tobacco, alcohol, and drug abuse prevention, he is the developer of the Life Skills Training approach to drug abuse prevention, which is widely viewed as the most effective school-based prevention program currently available. He is the author or co-author of more than 120 scientific papers and book chapters and has given invited addresses at conferences throughout the United States and Europe. Dr. Botvin has served as a consultant or advisor to the World Health Organization and numerous local, state, and federal agencies, including the National Institute on Drug Abuse, the Office of National Drug Control Policy, the Center for Substance Abuse Prevention, the National Cancer Institute, the U.S. Department of Education, and the National Centers for Disease Control and Prevention. In 1994, he received the Federal Bureau of Investigation's national demand reduction award for excellence in drug abuse prevention and in 1995 he received a MERIT award from the National Institute of Drug Abuse.

Steven Schinke, PhD, is Professor in the School of Social Work at Columbia University in New York, New York, where he teaches research methods to doctoral students. Before joining Columbia in 1986, he was a faculty member of the University of Washington School of Social Work. His research focuses on prevention training, with an emphasis on substance abuse and minority culture adolescents. At present, he is Principal Investigator of research studies to develop and test preventive interventions aimed at tobacco and alcohol use among inner-city youth. The author of more than 170 articles on preventive interventions and skills training for adolescents, Dr. Schinke is a consulting editor to *Addictive Behaviors, Behavioral Medicine Abstracts, Children and Youth Services Review,* the *Journal of Adolescent Research,* the *Journal of Family Violence,* the *Journal of Social Service Research,* and *Research on Social Work Practice.*

Introduction

Gilbert J. Botvin
Steven Schinke

THE RETURN OF AN OLD PROBLEM

The problem of drug abuse has been with us since before the psychedelic sixties. After peaking in the late 1970s and early 1980s, drug use among our nation's youth declined for about a decade before bottoming out in the early 1990s. Since then, it has increased at an alarming rate (Johnston, O'Malley, & Bachman, 1995). The problem is particularly keen for junior and senior high school students among whom there has been a sharp increase in marijuana use among eighth, tenth, and twelfth graders as well as an increase for all three grade levels in the use of cigarettes, stimulants, LSD, and inhalants. For marijuana, lifetime use has nearly tripled since 1992 among eighth graders, has nearly doubled for tenth graders, and has increased by 50% for twelfth graders. Although not as dramatic, similar increases have occurred for other substances. The upward trend in drug use appears to be relatively broad, including adolescents from different age groups, social classes, geographic regions, and racial/ethnic groups. Concern that these increases in adolescent drug use may herald the beginning of a new drug epidemic provides renewed impetus for increasing knowledge concerning the causes of drug use and effective methods for preventing it.

DRUG USE AMONG MINORITY YOUTH

Since 1991, when racial/ethnic differences were included in the national estimates for secondary school students, black youths have reported the

[Haworth co-indexing entry note]: "Introduction." Botvin, Gilbert J., and Steven Schinke. Co-published simultaneously in *Journal of Child & Adolescent Substance Abuse* (The Haworth Press, Inc.) Vol. 6, No. 1, 1997, pp. 1-3; and: *The Etiology and Prevention of Drug Abuse Among Minority Youth* (ed: Gilbert J. Botvin, and Steven Schinke) The Haworth Press, Inc., 1997, pp. 1-3. Single or multiple copies of this article are available for a fee from The Haworth Document Delivery Service [1-800-342-9678, 9:00 a.m. - 5:00 p.m. (EST). E-mail address: getinfo@haworth.com].

lowest prevalence estimates for all drugs mentioned in survey, whereas Hispanic youth have reported the highest lifetime, annual, and recent 30-day prevalence. A somewhat different picture emerges, however, from the National Household Survey on Drug Abuse (National Institute on Drug Abuse [NIDA], 1991) which lumps together a broader range inclusive of 12 year olds through 17 year olds. In this survey, which relies on face-to-face interviews, prevalence estimates for marijuana use in the past year are largely the same for blacks (10.4%), whites (10.3%), and Hispanics (9.4%). More recent data from the 1993 survey shows that annual illicit drug use among Hispanics has increased from 13.3% to 17.6%, and is the highest level among the three largest race groups. Whites are second at 13.5%, followed by blacks (11.0%) for any illicit drug use in the past year (Substance Abuse and Mental Health Services Administration, 1994).

THE NEED FOR RESEARCH WITH MINORITY YOUTH

One of the most significant gaps in the literature on drug abuse concerns the conspicuous absence of high quality research concerning the etiology and prevention of drug abuse among minority youth. The two largest ethnic minority groups in the United States, African-Americans and Hispanics, are at significant risk for drug abuse and drug-related problems (Botvin, Schinke, & Orlandi, 1995). A major limitation of the existing literature is that it consists of studies conducted with predominantly white, middle-class adolescents. Additional research is needed to better understand the role of ethnic factors in the etiology of drug abuse as well as to better understand the etiology of drug abuse among disadvantaged, inner-city, minority youth. Additional research is also warranted to increase our understanding of the extent to which prevention approaches developed and tested on white youth are effective with minority youth or to identify new approaches tailored to minority youth.

OVERVIEW OF THE SPECIAL VOLUME

The papers contained in this special volume provide important new information concerning drug use among minority youth. Some of the papers focus on issues related to etiology while others are more related to prevention. These papers evolved out of a program of research funded by the National Institute on Drug Abuse under the umbrella of a center grant to Cornell University Medical College's Institute for Prevention Research concerning drug abuse prevention with multiethnic youth.

Although considerable research has been conducted in recent years, most has been conducted in school settings, has involved white, middle-class populations, and has focussed on cigarette smoking. The paper by Botvin and his colleagues provides data from a study testing the generalizability to inner-city minority youth of a prevention approach previously found to be effective on white youth. The effectiveness of this prevention approach is tested in terms of its impact on several measures of drug use, polydrug use, and behavioral intentions as well as hypothesized mediating variables. The paper by Scheier and his colleagues examines the role of ethnic identity as a moderator of psychosocial risk for alcohol and marijuana use. Following this is a paper by Schinke and his colleagues that is designed to provide the conceptual foundation for extending prevention methods found effective in school settings to the community. The paper discusses relevant theory, principles of prevention, and specific strategies along with a review of the results of studies testing community-based prevention approaches. The remaining two papers address issues related to the etiology of drug abuse in minority populations. The paper by Williams and his colleagues focuses on a sample of inner-city minority youth living in public housing developments and contrasts to similar youth living in conventional inner-city housing to determine the extent to which the conditions of public housing may affect the etiology of drug abuse. Finally, Diaz and her colleagues present the results of research examining the factors promoting drug abuse in youth living in shelters for homeless families. All five of these papers provide information likely to be useful in developing more effective preventative interventions for inner-city, minority youth. Yet, while they represent an important advance in knowledge about the etiology and prevention of drug abuse in minority populations, considerably more work remains to be done.

REFERENCES

Botvin, G.J., Schinke, S., & Orlandi, M.A. (1995). *Drug Abuse Prevention with Multiethnic Youth*. Thousand Oaks, CA: Sage Publications.

Johnston, L.D., O'Malley, P.M., & Bachman, J.G. (1995). *National Survey Results on Drug Use from the Monitoring the Future Study, 1975-1994. Volume I Secondary School Students*. Rockville, MD: US Department of Health and Human Services.

National Institute on Drug Abuse (1991). *National Household Survey on Drug Abuse: Population Estimates 1991*. Rockville, MD: US Department of Health and Human Services.

Substance Abuse and Mental Health Services Administration (1994). *National Household Survey on Drug Abuse: Population Estimates 1993*. Rockville, MD: US Department of Health and Human Services.

School-Based Drug Abuse Prevention with Inner-City Minority Youth

Gilbert J. Botvin
Jennifer A. Epstein
Eli Baker
Tracy Diaz
Michelle Ifill-Williams

SUMMARY. This study tested the effectiveness of a drug abuse prevention intervention with a predominantly minority sample of seventh-grade students (N = 721) in 7 urban schools in New York City. The drug abuse prevention curriculum teaches social resistance skills within the context of a broader intervention promoting general personal and social competence and implemented by regular classroom teachers. Results indicated that this approach was effective on several behavioral measures of current drug use including measures of polydrug use and on intention measures relevant to future drug

Gilbert J. Botvin, PhD, Jennifer A. Epstein, PhD, Eli Baker, PhD, Tracy Diaz, MA, and Michelle Ifill-Williams, MSW, MPH, are affiliated with the Institute for Prevention Research, Cornell University Medical College, 411 East 69th Street, New York, NY 10021.

Address correspondence to Gilbert J. Botvin, PhD, Institute for Prevention Research, Department of Public Health, Cornell University Medical College, 411 East 69th Street, New York, NY 10021.

This research was supported by funds from the National Institute for Drug Abuse (P50DA7656).

Portions of this research were presented in a symposium at the 103rd Annual Meeting of the American Psychological Association in August 1995.

use. Furthermore, there was some evidence for factors presumed to mediate the effects of this type of intervention (normative expectations and refusal skills). The significance of these findings is that they provide further support for the generalizability to a minority inner-city adolescent population of an approach previously found to be effective with white middle-class adolescent populations. In addition, this is the first time that effects have been shown with inner-city minority youth for the use of multiple drugs. *[Article copies available for a fee from The Haworth Document Delivery Service: 1-800-342-9678. E-mail address: getinfo@haworth.com]*

KEYWORDS. Adolescent Drug Use, Prevention, School-Based, Minority Youth

INTRODUCTION

Drug abuse has been recognized for more than three decades to be a serious public health threat. Examination of the most recent national survey data of adolescent drug use (Johnston, O'Malley and Bachman, 1995) reveals two disturbing facts. First, the prevalence of drug use among our nation's youth is at an unacceptably high level. Second, these data also show a reversal of the downward trend in the use of many drugs which had been underway throughout most of the 1980s and a steady increase in drug use for the past three years. This provides a new impetus for the development of effective approaches to drug abuse prevention. Unfortunately, economically disadvantaged inner-city minority adolescents remain an understudied population in terms of both the etiology and prevention of drug use. Yet these adolescents may be at increased risk for drug use (Oetting and Beauvais, 1990) or developing drug-related problems later in life (Kandel, 1995).

While drug abuse prevention programs focusing on the psychosocial factors that appear to promote and sustain drug use have been demonstrated to be effective with white middle-class adolescents, there has been surprisingly little research extending these findings to inner-city minority youth. Literature reviews (Botvin, 1986; Goodstadt, 1986; Flay, 1985; Hansen, 1992) and meta-analytic studies (Bangert-Drowns, 1988; Bruvold and Rundall, 1988; Tobler, 1986) have consistently supported the superiority of prevention approaches that target social influences either alone or with skills training over more traditional information dissemination approaches. These psychosocial approaches to drug abuse prevention are based on social learning theory (Bandura, 1977), communications theory

(McGuire, 1964), and problem behavior theory (Jessor and Jessor, 1977). From this perspective, drug use initiation is viewed as a consequence of the interplay of interpersonal and intrapersonal factors. Drug use is conceptualized as a behavior that is learned through a process of modeling and reinforcement from various social influences including peers, family members, and the media. Vulnerability to these influences is determined by domain-specific cognitions, attitudes, and expectations, as well as the availability of skills for coping with drug use offers and other life situations confronting adolescents. Prevention approaches that are based on this formulation typically emphasize increasing students' awareness of the social influences promoting drug use, modifying normative expectations concerning drug use, and teaching skills for resisting drug use pressures (e.g., Pentz, Dwyer, MacKinnon, Flay, Hansen, Wang and Johnson, 1989). Other programs also include the teaching of personal competence and social skills (e.g., Botvin, Baker, Dusenbury, Tortu and Botvin, 1990), in an effort to decrease motivation to use drugs and increase vulnerability to drug use social influences.

A major weakness of the prevention literature is that most of the existing research has been conducted with predominantly white middle-class adolescent populations. Despite the success of the most promising psychosocial approaches to drug abuse prevention, there is considerable skepticism about their potential generalizability to minority adolescents. Yet, these programs appear to address important risk factors for smoking, alcohol, and marijuana use among inner-city minority youth. Moreover, there is at least preliminary support for the effectiveness of these approaches from several small-scale pilot studies (Botvin, Batson et al., 1989; Botvin, Dusenbury et al., 1989) and one large-scale study (Botvin, Dusenbury et al., 1992) that targeted minority adolescents. Still more research is necessary to increase our understanding of what works with inner-city minority youth.

A second limitation is that most studies have been limited to cigarette smoking. Additional research is needed to determine the generalizability of current prevention approaches on other drugs. Another limitation of previous prevention research is the paucity of information concerning the mediating mechanisms of effective prevention approaches. Although some studies have attempted to address this issue (Botvin, Dusenbury, Baker et al., 1992), more research is needed to understand how effective prevention approaches work in order to further improve prevention models and advance prevention theory.

The purpose of the current study was to test a cognitive-behavioral approach to drug abuse prevention to (1) determine its effectiveness with inner-city minority youth for preventing cigarette smoking, (2) determine its impact on other forms of drug use including polydrug use, and (3) determine its impact on hypothesized mediating variables.

METHOD

Overview

The seven participating junior high schools were assigned to either (1) receive a promising psychosocial drug abuse prevention program or (2) serve as a "standard care" control condition. The students in the control schools received the program that was normally in place at New York City schools. Informed and consenting seventh-grade students participated in pretest measurements. Approximately three months later, the students completed posttest measurements. Measurements consisted of responses obtained from one of two versions of a questionnaire and a carbon monoxide breath test. The two versions of the questionnaire had overlapping core items and sections that differed from one another. These later sections were also reversed to obtain higher completion rates.

Sample

A total of 833 seventh-grade students in seven schools completed the pretest questionnaire. Of the students who participated in the pretest, 721 (87%) provided data at both the pretest and posttest. The sample was 53% girls and 47% boys. The age of the students ranged from 11 to 15 and their average age was 12.6 (SD = .65). The ethnic-racial composition was 25.8% African-American, 69.6% Hispanic, .7% White, 1.4% Asian, 1.5% Native American, and 1.0% other. Among African-Americans, 70.8% described themselves as African-American, 21.7% described themselves as Caribbean/West Indian, and the rest described themselves as African (.8%) or other (6.7%). Of the Hispanics, the students were predominantly Puerto Rican (47.5%) and Dominican (41.6%) with low proportions of Cubans (.6%), Colombians (.4%), Mexican (.4%), Ecuadorian (2.3%) and other combinations (7.1%). The family structure was 37.3% mother-only household, 35% mother and father household, 12.1% mother and stepfather household, 1.4% father-only household, 1.4% father and stepmother household, 1.2% foster parents household, 5.1% grandparent household, and 6.5% other composition. The sample was composed of economically disadvantaged youth from predominantly low socioeconomic status families: 76.2%

of the students indicated that they receive free lunch from school and 2.4% buy lunch at school for a reduced price, 9.9% of the students either bring their lunch from home or go home for lunch, 1.3% pay the full price for school lunch, and 10.2% buy lunch outside of school.

Procedure

After their school had been assigned to either treatment or control conditions, all students provided pretest data, participated in either the 15-session psychosocial prevention program or the program normally provided in the control schools, and provided posttest data approximately three months after the pretest. Data were collected following a detailed protocol similar to those used in previous research (e.g., Botvin, Schinke, Epstein and Diaz, 1994). Self-reported drug use behavior was assessed by questionnaire along with relevant cognitive, attitudinal, and personality variables. Students were assured about the confidentiality of their responses and unique identification codes were utilized rather than names to permit linkage of pretest and posttest responses and emphasize the confidential nature of the survey. Questionnaires were administered during a regular 40-minute classroom period by a team of three to five data collectors who were members of the same ethnic-minority groups as the participating students. Carbon monoxide (CO) breath samples were also collected at both the pretest and posttest to enhance the validity of self-report data utilizing a variant of the procedure developed by Evans and his colleagues (Evans, Hansen and Mittlemark, 1977). Although the collection of CO samples is most directly related to cigarette smoking, prior research suggests that these procedures can also enhance the validity of adolescents' self reports of alcohol and marijuana use (E. Botvin, G. J. Botvin, Renick, Filazzola and Allegrante, 1984).

Prevention Program

The preventive intervention taught drug resistance skills, anti-drug norms and material designed to facilitate the development of important personal and social skills. The goal of the prevention program was to provide adolescents with the requisite knowledge and skills for resisting social influences to use cigarettes, alcohol and drugs as well as to reduce potential motivations to use alcohol and drugs by increasing general personal competence (Botvin, 1982). As a consequence, the curriculum was designed to address the major cognitive, attitudinal, psychological, and social factors that are either empirically or conceptually related to tobacco, alcohol, and drug use.

More specifically, the prevention program teaches students cognitive-behavioral skills for building self-esteem, resisting advertising pressure, managing anxiety, communicating effectively, developing personal relationships, and asserting one's rights. These skills are taught using a combination of teaching techniques including group discussion, demonstration, modeling, behavioral rehearsal, feedback and reinforcement, and behavioral "homework" assignments for out-of-class practice. In addition to teaching skills for the enhancement of generic personal and social competence, the program teaches problem-specific skills related to drug use. For example, students are taught the application of general assertive skills in situations in which they might experience direct interpersonal pressure to smoke, drink, or use drugs. Moreover, unlike traditional prevention approaches, only minimal information concerning the long-term health consequences of drug use is provided. Instead, information hypothesized to be more salient to adolescents and relevant to prevention is provided including information concerning the immediate negative consequences of use, the decreasing social acceptability of use, and the actual prevalence rates among adults and adolescents. Material is also provided to reinforce nondrug use norms and modify pro-drug use normative expectations.

Over the past several years, this approach has been revised for use with minority youth in other studies (Botvin, Dusenbury, Baker, James-Ortiz and Kerner, 1989; Botvin, Batson, Witts-Vitale, Bess, Baker and Dusenbury, 1989; Botvin, Dusenbury, Baker, James-Ortiz, Botvin and Kerner, 1992). Although the underlying prevention strategy has remained constant for the different ethnic groups, modifications were made with respect to reading level, examples used to illustrate program content, and suggested situations for behavioral exercises. Intervention materials included a teacher's manual with detailed lesson-plans, student handouts, and video material demonstrating the personal and social skills being taught in the prevention program by same-age minority adolescents. The prevention program was implemented by regular classroom teachers who had attended a one-day teacher training workshop. The purpose of the workshop was to familiarize the teachers with the content of the prevention program and the rationale for the cognitive-behavioral skills training prevention strategy (Tortu and Botvin, 1989).

Measures

The variables included in this study were assessed using two questionnaire versions (version A and version B) that were randomly distributed to students in each class so that each questionnaire version was completed by about half the sample. In addition, the order of items/sections was modified in version B of the questionnaire starting with the later sections of the questionnaire to maximize the amount of information collected on each variable assessed and to minimize data loss due to fatigue, boredom, or inadequate time. Both questionnaires included the same 54 core items. Version A consisting of 133 items was completed by 347 students and version B consisting of 124 items was completed by 374 students.

Many of the measures used were derived from well-known and widely-used instruments. These measures have been used in previous prevention studies with white adolescents and minority adolescents. The questionnaire assessed current drug use and intentions for drug use in the future. The questionnaire items measured cognitive, attitudinal, and skills variables associated with the initiation of drug use. Although all measures were self-reported, the confidential nature of the data being collected was emphasized by data collectors to minimize problems related to validity. In addition, correlations between the drug use measures and related measures (e.g., friends' drug use) were high suggesting high construct validity. The questionnaire also included demographic items and measures concerning the perceived prevalence of drug use by adults and peers. In addition, new skills measures were developed to reflect the content of the prevention program. During the instrument development phase of this study, the questionnaire was administered to minority adolescents in focus groups. Based on feedback from these focus groups, changes were made to ensure the suitability of the measures and their working for the target population. Where appropriate, reliabilities (Cronbach's alpha) calculated from the pretest sample for the scales are indicated in parentheses in the description that follows. Only those scales retained after preliminary analyses and relevant to the evaluation of the intervention are included.

Demographic data. Data concerning the characteristics of the participants were collected using standard survey items concerning gender, age, family structure, race and ethnicity, socioeconomic status (receive free or reduced school lunch), religion, academic performance, absenteeism, and educational aspirations.

Drug use. Cigarette smoking was assessed using an 11-point smoking index anchored by "never smoked" (1) and "a pack or more a day" (11). Alcohol use was measured in three ways. Drinking frequency for alcoholic beverages was assessed using a nine-point drinking index anchored by "never tried them" (1) and "more than once a day" (9). Amount of alcohol consumed per drinking occasion was assessed using a six-point scale ranging from "I don't drink" (1) to "more than six drinks" (6). The frequency of getting drunk was measured using a nine-point drunkenness index anchored by "I don't drink" (1) and "more than once a day" (9). Marijuana use was assessed using a nine-point marijuana index anchored by "never tried it" (1) and "more than once a day" (9).

Polydrug use. Measures of multiple drug use were created based on the responses to the smoking index, drinking index, and marijuana index. For each index, two variables were constructed: ever use and current use. Specifically, the ever use variables were dichotomized into two categories: students who had never tried the drug and students who had tried the drug. The current use variables were dichotomized into two categories: students who never used the drug or used it less than once a month and students who used the drug once a month or more. These ever use and current use variables were combined to form two composite measures of polydrug use to identify individuals who had ever used all three gateway drugs or were currently using them.

Behavioral intention. Behavioral intentions to use six types of drugs (cigarettes, beer or wine, hard liquor, marijuana or hashish, cocaine/crack and other hard drugs) within the next year were measured on five-point scales anchored by "definitely not" (1) and "definitely will" (5).

Normative expectations. Normative expectations related to drug use (smoke cigarettes, drink beer or wine, smoke marijuana, use cocaine/crack, use other hard drugs) were assessed in terms of: (1) perceived prevalence of drug use among peers (peer norms), and (2) perceived prevalence of drug use among adults (adult norms). For each drug, peer norms and adult norms were measured on five-point scales anchored by "none" (1) and "all or almost all" (5).

Attitudes toward drug use. Respondents' attitudes about smoking, drinking, marijuana, and cocaine or other drugs, the characteristics of users and the perceived social benefits of using these drugs were assessed by four parallel measures. The smoking items were derived from the *Teenager's Self-Test: Cigarette Smoking* (U.S. Public Health Service, 1974). Parallel items were developed for alcohol, marijuana, and cocaine or other drugs. Five items were used to assess attitudes about smoking (alpha = .85), alcohol (alpha = .86), marijuana (alpha = .91), and cocaine or other drugs (alpha = .90). Responses were indicated on five-point Likert scales anchored by "strongly disagree" (1) and "strongly agree" (5).

Social competence. Students were also assessed with respect to their use of: decision making (6 items; alpha = .72), advertising influences (6 items; alpha = .80), anxiety reduction (6 items; alpha = .77), and communication (4 items; alpha = .67). Assertiveness was assessed using an empirically reduced version of the *Gambrill and Richey* (1975) *Assertion Inventory*. The responses were rated on five-point Likert scales anchored by "never" (1) and "always" (5). Two subscales were created: refusal skills assertiveness and social assertiveness. Refusal skills assertiveness consisted of five items related to saying "no" to drug use and to doing something that you don't want to do (alpha = .87). Social assertiveness consisted of five items measuring assertiveness in social interactions such as saying what you believe even if others disagree and starting a conversation with someone you want to know better (alpha = .76).

Data Analysis

Data analyses were conducted according to the following procedures. First, the pretest comparability of the two conditions (prevention and control) for the demographic variables and the drug use variables was determined. Then, the effectiveness of the intervention was tested using a series of General Linear Model (GLM) analyses. These analyses were conducted for students present at both the pretest and posttest. Pretest scores were used as covariates in all the GLM analyses. As in previous research (e.g., Botvin et al., 1995) with this approach, one-tailed significance tests were used for the analyses of intervention effects as warranted by the uni-directional nature of hypothesized effects, as well as the results of previous research using similar prevention approaches.

RESULTS

Pretest Equivalence

Treatment and control conditions were compared on demographic and behavioral variables to determine the comparability of groups at the pretest. A series of crosstabulations were conducted to test the pretest equivalence of the demographic variables by condition. There were no significant differences between conditions for gender, free lunch, or family structure. There were differences between conditions based on race/ethnicity, with a lower proportion of Hispanic students and a greater proportion of African-American students in the control condition (57% Hispanic, 37% African-American) than in the prevention (76% Hispanic, 20% African-American) group. However, race/ethnicity was not related to any of the pretest drug use variables. The comparison of the prevention and control conditions with respect to the primary behavioral outcome variables from the pretest indicated that there were no significant differences; therefore the conditions were comparable at the pretest.

Current Drug Use and Behavioral Intentions

Univariate GLM ANCOVAs were conducted for each of the individual drug use, multiple drug use, and future intention dependent variables. The results of these analyses including the adjusted posttest means are summarized in Table 1. Significant treatment effects were found for all of the five individual drug use behavior variables and both of the multiple drug use measures. As shown in Table 1, the students in the prevention condition smoked cigarettes significantly less often (p < .01), drank alcohol significantly less often (p < .01), consumed significantly less alcohol (p < .001), became drunk significantly less often (p < .05), and smoked marijuana less frequently (p < .05) than the students in the control group. Most interestingly, both the level of ever use of multiple drugs (p < .0001) and current (monthly) use of multiple drugs (p < .01) were lower in the prevention condition than the control condition. Future intentions to smoke cigarettes (p < .01), drink beer or wine (p < .01), smoke marijuana (p < .05), or use cocaine (p = .06) within the next year were lower in the prevention group relative to the control group.

TABLE 1. Adjusted Posttest Means for Substance Use by Condition

	Prevention		Control				
Variable	Mean	SE	Mean	SE	F	df	p
Behavioral Measures							
Smoking Index	1.63	.05	1.87	.06	9.27	1,710	.0012
Drinking Index	1.73	.05	2.00	.07	8.69	1,696	.0017
Drinking Amount	1.43	.03	1.62	.05	10.68	1,684	.0006
Drunkenness	1.33	.04	1.49	.06	4.95	1,689	.0133
Marijuana Index	1.16	.03	1.26	.05	2.79	1,703	.0477
Multiple Substances							
Ever Use Measure	.92	.03	1.09	.04	10.85	1,718	.0001
Current Use Measure	.15	.02	.24	.03	6.54	1,718	.0054
Intention to Use Within Next Year							
Cigarettes	1.55	.04	1.72	.05	6.87	1,699	.0045
Beer/Wine	1.78	.04	1.98	.06	6.93	1,685	.0044
Liquor	1.24	.03	1.28	.04	.77	1,685	.1903
Marijuana	1.13	.02	1.20	.03	2.81	1,687	.0471
Cocaine	1.02	.01	1.05	.02	2.53	1,689	.0562
Other Drugs	1.03	.01	1.05	.02	.93	1,685	.1672

Note: Significance levels are based on one-tailed tests.

Impact on Hypothesized Mediating Variables

A series of ANCOVAs was computed to determine the impact of the intervention on the hypothesized mediating variables. Table 2 presents the results of the ANCOVAs for the attitudes, normative expectations, and skills measures. Significant differences were found between the prevention and control conditions for normative expectations regarding drug use (i.e., perceived drug use by adults and peers). The prevention group had significantly lower normative expectations than the control group concerning adult smoking ($p < .001$), peer smoking ($p < .01$), adult drinking ($p < .01$), peer drinking ($p < .0001$), peer marijuana use ($p < .01$), adult cocaine use ($p < .01$), peer cocaine use ($p < .05$), other drug use by adults ($p < .05$), and other drug use by peers ($p < .01$). Finally, students in the

TABLE 2. Adjusted Posttest Means for Attitudes, Expectations and Skills by Condition

Variable	Prevention		Control		F	df	p
	Mean	SE	Mean	SE			
Substance Use Attitudes							
Anti-Smoking	87.32	1.05	87.74	1.44	.06	1,269	.4064
Anti-Drinking	90.56	1.03	88.82	1.40	1.00	1,271	.1594
Anti-Marijuana	92.40	0.96	91.22	1.29	.53	1,266	.2331
Anti-Drug	94.20	0.88	94.37	1.20	.00	1,262	.4760
Normative Expectations							
Adult Smoking	3.59	0.05	3.86	0.07	10.96	1,686	.0005
Peer Smoking	2.84	0.05	3.07	0.07	8.66	1,694	.0017
Adult Drinking	3.59	0.05	3.80	0.07	6.36	1,684	.0060
Peer Drinking	2.65	0.05	3.00	0.07	16.52	1,688	.0001
Adult Marijuana Use	2.64	0.05	2.76	0.08	1.80	1,674	.0900
Peer Marijuana Use	2.38	0.05	2.64	0.07	8.44	1,675	.0019
Adult Cocaine	2.37	0.05	2.61	0.07	6.67	1,673	.0050
Peer Cocaine	1.84	0.05	2.00	0.06	4.34	1,678	.0188
Adult Other Drugs	2.32	0.06	2.53	0.08	4.88	1,675	.0138
Peer Other Drugs	1.82	0.05	2.01	0.06	6.13	1,681	.0068
Skills Use							
Decision-Making	61.68	1.38	58.85	1.92	1.43	1,297	.1166
Advertising	55.06	1.76	56.17	2.44	.14	1,281	.3561
Anxiety Reduction	43.15	1.55	46.46	2.18	1.53	1,279	.1086
Communication	63.53	1.44	62.22	2.03	.28	1,259	.3002
Refusal Assertiveness	88.75	1.48	83.02	2.03	5.24	1,274	.0114
Social Assertiveness	67.03	1.40	67.00	1.93	.00	1,276	.4938

Note: Significance levels are based on one-tailed tests.

prevention condition were significantly more likely to use refusal skills ($p < .05$) than the students in the control group.

DISCUSSION

The results of this study provide further support for the effectiveness of a psychosocial approach to drug abuse prevention with inner-city minority adolescents. Past research demonstrated the effectiveness of this approach in smoking prevention for African-American adolescents (Botvin, Batson et al., 1989) and Hispanic adolescents (Botvin, Dusenbury et al., 1989; Botvin, Dusenbury et al., 1992). Moreover, a recent study conducted with minority students supported this approach in lowering intentions to drink alcohol in the future relative to a control group (Botvin et al., 1994).

Past research conducted with predominantly white middle-class populations showed that psychosocial approaches can prevent smoking, alcohol use, and marijuana use (e.g., Botvin et al., 1990). However, this is the first time that lower levels of smoking, alcohol, and marijuana use have been demonstrated in a sample of inner-city minority adolescents who participated in this type of prevention program. Furthermore, the results concerning intentions to use cocaine in the future suggest that this approach may generalize to other illicit drugs. Since experience with other illicit drugs typically occurs after use of a licit drug and marijuana (Kandel and Yamaguchi, 1993; Kandel et al., 1992), it is conceivable that prevention effects for other illicit drug use might emerge over a longer-term follow-up period with minority youth as they have in research with middle-class white youth (Botvin et al., 1995). In another new finding with this population, the results of this study also revealed that the psychosocial drug abuse prevention approach tested in this study influenced polydrug use. Specifically, experimentation and current use of multiple drugs (cigarettes, alcohol, and marijuana) were lower in the prevention group relative to the control group.

As predicted, the students who received the psychosocial intervention had lower normative expectations concerning the various drugs (cigarettes, alcohol, marijuana, cocaine, and other drugs) than students in the control group. This replicates the findings of earlier evaluations of this approach for smoking with minority youth (Botvin, Batson et al., 1989; Botvin, Dusenbury et al., 1989) including a large-scale study that demonstrated that normative expectations mediated the impact of the intervention on cigarette smoking (Botvin et al., 1992). Therefore, this series of studies suggests that modifying normative expectations plays an important role in preventing drug use. However, the results of a recent study testing the type of intervention utilized in this study against one which was designed to change drug-related knowledge and normative expectations (Botvin, Schinke, Epstein and Diaz, 1994) suggest that modifying normative expectations is an important but not an essential ingredient in effective prevention approaches. Indeed, the results of the current study also provide evidence for the importance of teaching refusal skills for resisting offers to use drugs.

It should also be noted, however, that this study has several limitations. First, this study involved a small number of students from a small number of schools. Obviously because this was a small-scale study, it was not possible to determine the relative effectiveness of this type of prevention strategy for the various subgroups in the sample. A larger-scale study is currently underway which will address this issue by testing the efficacy of this approach for Hispanics and African-American youth separately. Another potential limitation of this and other similar studies is the reliance on self-report data. To address this, CO data were also collected using procedures which have been found to increase the accuracy of self-reports (Evans, Hansen and Mittlemark, 1977). Moreover, the intercorrelations among the various drug use measures and other related measures provide additional support for the validity of these data.

The findings from this study are encouraging and should facilitate further development of effective approaches to drug abuse prevention for both white and minority youth. The psychosocial prevention approach tested in this study produced an impact on all of the behavioral drug use measures, including two based on polydrug use. Normative expectations and refusal assertiveness were implicated as important mediating mechanisms in the effectiveness of this type of psychosocial approach. Further research is necessary to elucidate the factors promoting drug use among minority adolescents and identify effective strategies for preventing both gateway drug use and the use of illicit drugs other than marijuana.

REFERENCES

Bandura, A. (1977). *Social learning theory.* Englewood Cliffs, NJ: Prentice Hall.

Bangert-Drowns, R.L. (1988). The effects of school-based substance abuse education—A meta-analysis. *Journal of Drug Education, 18*(31), 243-265.

Botvin, E.M., Botvin, G.J., Renick, N.L., Filazzola, A.D., & Allegrante, J.P. (1984). Adolescents' self-reports of tobacco, alcohol, and marijuana use: Examining the comparability of video tape, cartoon, and verbal bogus pipeline procedures. *Psychological Reports, 55,* 379-386.

Botvin, G.J. (1982). Broadening the focus of smoking prevention strategies. In: Coates, T., Peterson, A., Perry, C., eds. *Promoting Adolescent Health: A Dialogue on Research and Practice.* New York: Academic Press.

Botvin, G.J. (1986). Substance abuse prevention research: Recent developments and future directions. *Journal of School Health, 56,* 369-386.

Botvin, G.J., Baker, E., Dusenbury, L., Botvin, E.M., & Diaz, T. (1995). Long-term follow-up results of a randomized drug abuse prevention trial in a White middle-class population. *Journal of the American Medical Association, 273*(14), 1106-1112.

Botvin, G.J., Baker, E., Dusenbury, L., Tortu, S., & Botvin, E.M. (1990). Preventing adolescent drug abuse through a multimodal cognitive-behavioral approach: Results of a three-year study. *Journal of Consulting and Clinical Psychology, 58*(4), 437-446.

Botvin, G.J., Batson, H., Witts-Vitale, S., Bess, V., Baker, E., & Dusenbury, L. (1989). A psychosocial approach to smoking prevention for urban Black youth. *Public Health Reports, 104,* 573-582.

Botvin, G.J., Dusenbury, L., Baker, E., James-Ortiz, S., Botvin, E.M., & Kerner, J. (1992). Smoking prevention among urban minority youth: Assessing effects on outcome and mediating variables. *Health Psychology, 11*(5), 290-299.

Botvin, G.J., Dusenbury, L., Baker, E., James-Ortiz, S., & Kerner, J. (1989). A skills training approach to smoking prevention among hispanic youth. *Journal of Behavioral Medicine, 12,* 279-296.

Botvin, G.J., Schinke, S.P., Epstein, J.A., & Diaz, T. (1994). Effectiveness of culturally-focused and generic skills training approaches to alcohol and drug abuse prevention among minority youths. *Psychology of Addictive Behaviors, 8,* 116-127.

Bruvold, W.H., & Rundall, T.G. (1988). A meta-analysis and theoretical review of school based tobacco and alcohol intervention programs. *Psychology and Health, 2,* 53-78.

Evans, R.I., Hansen, W.B., & Mittlemark, M.B. (1977). Increasing the validity of self-reports of smoking behavior in children. *Journal of Applied Psychology, 62,* 521-523.

Flay, B.R. (1985). Psychosocial approaches to smoking prevention: A review of findings. *Health Psychology, 4,* 449-488.

Gambrill, E.D., & Richey, C.A. (1975). An assertion inventory for use in assessment and research. *Behavior Therapy, 6,* 550-561.

Goodstadt, M.S. (1986). Alcohol education research and practice: A logical analysis of the two realities. *Journal of Drug Education, 16,* 349-364.

Hansen, W.B. (1992). School based substance prevention: A review of the state-of-the-art in curriculum. *Health Education Research, 7,* 403-430.

Jessor, R., & Jessor, S.L. (1977). *Problem behavior and psychosocial development: A longitudinal study of youth.* New York: Academic Press.

Johnston, L.D., O'Malley, P.M., & Bachman, J.G. (1995). *National Survey Results on Drug Use from the Monitoring the Future Study, 1975-1994. Volume I Secondary School Students.* Rockville, MD: US Department of Health and Human Services.

Kandel, D.B. (1995). Ethnic differences in drug use: Patterns and paradoxes. In:

Botvin, G.J., Schinke, S., Orlandi, M.A., eds. *Drug Abuse Prevention with Multiethnic Youth*, (pp. 81-104). Thousand Oaks, CA: Sage.

Kandel, D., & Yamaguchi, K. (1993). From beer to crack: Developmental patterns of drug involvement. *American Journal of Public Health*, *83*(6), 851-855.

Kandel, D.B., Yamaguchi, K., & Chen, K. (1992). Stages of progression in drug involvement from adolescence to adulthood: Further evidence for the Gateway Theory. *Journal of Studies on Alcohol*, *53*, 447-457.

McGuire, W.J. (1964). Inducing resistance to persuasion: Some contemporary approaches. In: Berkowitz, L., ed. *Advances in Experimental Social Psychology*, (pp. 192-227). New York: Academic Press.

Oetting, E.R., & Beauvais, F. (1990). Adolescent drug use: Findings of national and local surveys. *Journal of Consulting and Clinical Psychology*, *58*, 385-394.

Pentz, M.A., Dwyer, J.H., MacKinnon, D.P., Flay, B.R., Hansen, W.B., Wang, E.Y., & Johnson, C.A. (1989). A multicommunity trial for primary prevention of adolescent drug abuse. Effects on drug prevalence. *Journal of the American Medical Association*, *261*, 3259-3266.

Tobler, N. (1986). Meta-analysis of 143 adolescent drug prevention programs: Quantitative outcome results of program participants compared to a control or comparison group. *J of Drug Issues*, *16*, 537-567.

Tortu, S., & Botvin, G.J. (1989). School-based smoking prevention: The teacher training process. *Preventive Medicine*, *18*, 280-289.

U.S. Public Health Service. (1974). *Teenager's self-test: Cigarette smoking.* Washington, DC: Centers for Disease Control: U.S. Public Health Service (DHEW Publication No. CDC 74-8723).

Ethnic Identity as a Moderator of Psychosocial Risk and Adolescent Alcohol and Marijuana Use: Concurrent and Longitudinal Analyses

Lawrence M. Scheier
Gilbert J. Botvin
Tracy Diaz
Michelle Ifill-Williams

SUMMARY. Studies of psychosocial risk and adolescent drug use among minority youth have been primarily descriptive in nature. This may be an unfortunate oversight, particularly because developmental studies indicate that cultural factors play an important role in the etiology of mental health problems. Utilizing data obtained from a sample of minority control students participating in a longitudinal

Lawrence M. Scheier, PhD, Gilbert J. Botvin, PhD, Tracy Diaz, MA, and Michelle Ifill-Williams, MSW, MPH, are affiliated with the Institute for Prevention Research, Cornell University Medical College, 411 East 69th Street, New York, NY 10021.

Address correspondence to Lawrence M. Scheier, Institute for Prevention Research, Department of Public Health, Cornell University Medical College, 411 East 69th Street, Kips Bay 201, New York, NY 10021. E-mail: lmscheie@mail.med.cornell.edu

Preparation of this article was partially supported by a research grant to Gilbert J. Botvin (P50DA-7656) and a FIRST Award to Lawrence M. Scheier (R29-DA08909-01) from the National Institute on Drug Abuse.

[Haworth co-indexing entry note]: "Ethnic Identity as a Moderator of Psychosocial Risk and Adolescent Alcohol and Marijuana Use: Concurrent and Longitudinal Analyses." Scheier, Lawrence M. et al. Co-published simultaneously in *Journal of Child & Adolescent Substance Abuse* (The Haworth Press, Inc.) Vol. 6, No. 1, 1997, pp. 21-47; and: *The Etiology and Prevention of Drug Abuse Among Minority Youth* (ed: Gilbert J. Botvin, and Steven Schinke) The Haworth Press, Inc., 1997, pp. 21-47. Single or multiple copies of this article are available for a fee from The Haworth Document Delivery Service [1-800-342-9678, 9:00 a.m. - 5:00 p.m. (EST). E-mail address: getinfo@haworth.com].

school-based drug prevention trial, we examined the role of ethnic identity as it moderates the relations between several domains of psychosocial risk and alcohol and marijuana use. A risk-factor methodology was used to construct additive risk indices that reflected key domains of a psychosocial model of deviant behavior. Results of cross-sectional analyses indicated that ethnic identity moderated the effects of alcohol-related expectancies, knowledge, and social skills for alcohol use; whereas ethnic identity moderated the effects of social influences, competence, and social skills for marijuana use. Results of longitudinal analyses found that ethnic identity moderated the effects of social skills on alcohol use and in some instances uniquely predicted both alcohol and marijuana use, controlling for risk. Findings are discussed in terms of the formative role of cultural factors as they shape vulnerability to adolescent alcohol and drug use. *[Article copies available for a fee from The Haworth Document Delivery Service: 1-800-342-9678. E-mail address: getinfo@haworth.com]*

KEYWORDS. Ethnic Identity, Drug Use, Alcohol Use, Adolescent

The search for key determinants of early-stage drug use has uncovered a wealth of information regarding the potential role of risk and protective factors (Hawkins, Catalano, and Miller, 1992; Petraitis, Flay, and Miller, 1995). Based on both cross-sectional and longitudinal studies, a common set of risk factors has emerged. Among the most prominent are social influences, interpersonal factors (e.g., poor communication and social skills), and intrapersonal factors (e.g., depression, low self-esteem, and poor competence).

Unfortunately, most of this research has largely focused on white populations. Relatively little research has examined the etiology of drug use among minority youth. More research is warranted to increase our understanding of the factors promoting drug use in minority populations, particularly because recent survey data obtained from both school (Johnston, O'Malley, and Bachman, 1995) and community samples (National Household Survey on Drug Abuse: NIDA, 1995) indicate that there is a growing similarity in drug use prevalence rates between minority and white youths. Moreover, the most recent census data show that African-American and Hispanic youth are the fastest growing segment of the U.S. population (U.S. Bureau of the Census, 1992).

Studies with minority youth must determine whether the same set of risk and protective factors promote drug use, whether these factors operate in the same manner with these youth, and the role played by cultural factors. To date, studies involving ethnic minority youth have not sufficiently examined the relationship between cultural factors and drug use (Collins, 1995; Trimble, 1995; Farrell, Danish, and Howard, 1992). Other studies that emphasize the need to understand cultural variables as they impact on drug use have either not included specific measures of ethnic identity (e.g., Dembo, Allen, Farrow, Schmeidler, and Burgos, 1985) or have rarely moved beyond the descriptive level of analysis in accounting for ethnic/racial differences in drug use (Bachman, Wallace, O'Malley, Johnston, Kurth, and Neighbors, 1991; Barnes and Welte, 1986; Dembo, Burgos, Des Jarlais, and Schmeidler, 1979; Flannery, Vazsonyi, Torquati, and Fridrich, 1994; Maddahian, Newcomb, and Bentler, 1985, 1988).

Among the few studies that have included ethnic or cultural identity in their etiological models, the findings have been mixed. For example, Trimble (1995) found that ethnic identity did not predict alcohol use, controlling for peer and adult influences in a sample of adolescent American Indians. Felix-Ortiz and Newcomb (1995) reported that cultural identity (i.e., language familiarity and cultural proficiency) differentially predicted patterns and variation in drug use among Hispanic adolescents. As these authors point out, a complicated picture emerges from both past and more recent studies of cultural identity and drug use, with some studies indicating a positive relationship and others indicating a negative one. Other research has demonstrated that ethnic or cultural identity plays an important role in the etiology of mental health problems (Phinney, Lochner, and Murphy, 1990) or is linked to self-esteem (Bautista de Domanico, Crawford, and De Wolfe, 1994; Whaley, 1993), personal and social development (Spencer, 1985), somatization patterns and health (Montgomery, 1992), and academic achievement and well-being (Arroyo and Zigler, 1995; Bernal, Saenz, and Knight, 1991).

One of the most crucial developmental tasks of adolescence is the formation and crystallization of an identity (Erikson, 1968). It is during this period that youth actively begin to construct a sense of who they are, formulate a plan for how they want to live their lives, and compare and contrast their skills and abilities with those of their closest friends and family. The synthesis of these diverse efforts culminates in the formation of a unified and coherent sense of personal identity. However, minority youth face the added challenge during this period of resolving issues of ethnic self-identification and ethnic validation (Aboud, 1987; Phinney, 1989, 1990). Phinney (1993) has suggested that minority adolescents "undergo a process of exploration and questioning about ethnicity in which they attempt to learn more about their culture and understand the implications of group membership" (p. 75). Failure to create a balance between ethnic and personal identity may result in feelings of cultural and personal inadequacy, marginality, and role confusion, all of which lead to alcohol and drug use as a means of coping with internal psychological pressures.

In recent years, a number of researchers have suggested that a risk factors approach best considers the problems of explanation and prediction when applied to adolescent drug use (Bry, 1983; Newcomb, Maddahian, and Bentler, 1986; Scheier and Newcomb, 1991). Rather than aiming to find the single best predictor that accounts for the largest portion of variance, a risk factors approach suggests that multiple risk factors, capturing multiple facets of psychosocial functioning, will better account for behavior. In keeping with this approach, risk is measured as a cumulative (additive) index that captures the relative amount of risk across a broad array of precursors and correlates of drug use. Using this approach, several studies successfully utilized a single index of relative risk to predict alcohol and other drug use (Bry, McKeon, and Pandina, 1986; Newcomb, Maddahian, and Bentler, 1986). Subsequently, Scheier and Newcomb (1991) demonstrated that multiple risk indices were needed to distinguish early stage (experimental) from more problematic drug use. In defining the utility of this approach, Newcomb (1992) proposed that a risk factor methodology closely adheres to a cumulative stress-resilience model, capturing multiple facets of several theoretical perspectives.

The paucity of data regarding the operation of developmental risk mechanisms in minority populations and evidence of increased drug use among minority youth point toward the need for additional etiology research. The current study was designed to increase our understanding of the etiology of drug use among minority youth and the role of cultural factors. Specifically, this study assessed the role of ethnic identity as a moderator of drug abuse risk using a risk factors methodology and seven distinct categories of risk. Each risk index closely corresponds with elements of the personality and environment systems (as well as different aspects of background-antecedent variables) of problem behavior theory (Jessor and Jessor, 1977). Outcome measures include both composite measures of alcohol (frequency, intensity, and drunkenness) and marijuana (frequency and intensity) use for both the cross-sectional analyses and longitudinal analyses. Drawing on findings from the social support literature (e.g., Cohen and Wills, 1985; Pearlin, Menaghan, Lieberman, and Mullan, 1981), we have conceptualized ethnic identity as a type of social support and hypothesize the moderator or buffering activity of ethnic identity to be analogous to the manner in which social support buffers against stress. High levels of ethnic identity are hypothesized to offset interpersonal and intrapersonal pressures to use drugs.

METHOD

Sample

Data for the current study were obtained as part of a prospective investigation of the etiology and prevention of drug use among inner-city youth. For the purposes of this study, a cohort of seventh grade minority youth attending nontreatment control schools served as subjects. Consistent with the focus of this study, the sample was restricted to African-American and Hispanic youth. A total of 1,815 youth met the inclusion criteria for the seventh grade cross-sectional sample (M = 12.96 years old, SD = 0.63) and 1,303 adolescents constituted the seventh/eighth grade longitudinal sample. The gender composition of the pretest minority sample was 52% female and the resultant sample was 60% African-American and 40% Hispanic. Thirty-seven percent of the sample reported living with both parents, whereas 39% reported living with their mother only, 11% with their mother and a step-parent, and the remaining percent reported living with some adult other than their parents. A majority of these youth reported receiving free lunch (66%), while a much smaller group (5%) received lunch at reduced prices or reported not eating at all (14%).

Procedure

Participating students provided data by surveys administered in the Fall of 1994 during the seventh grade (Time 1), three months later (Time 2), and a year later during the eighth grade (Time 3). Time 1 data were used for the cross-sectional analyses and the Time 1/Time 3 data were used for the longitudinal analyses. To preserve the confidentiality of the surveys and to facilitate longitudinal tracking, numerical identification codes were lithocoded on each survey. Passive consent was obtained from parents and the refusal rate for participation in the study was less than 1%. Data were collected by carefully trained field staff following standardized procedures for administering and collecting the questionnaires at each school (no questionnaires were handled by school personnel or teachers). A 40-minute classroom period was designated for data collection and aggressive tracking and follow-up procedures were used to gather data from absentee students.

Survey Instrument. Questionnaire items included measures of intra- and interpersonal functioning as well as a variety of attitudes, intentions, and behaviors related to alcohol, tobacco, and marijuana use. Behavioral measures included current frequency of use for alcohol (beer, wine, and hard liquor), cigarettes, and marijuana (including hashish). Item stems were worded: "About how often (if ever) do you," with responses ranging from "never" (1) to "more than once a day" (9). Using a similar stem and response format, one item assessed drunkenness: "How often do you drink until you get drunk" and one item tapped intensity of marijuana use: "How often do you smoke marijuana or hashish until you get high or stoned." Items assessing intensity were included for cigarettes: "If you smoke cigarettes, about how much do you usually smoke," responses ranging from "none at all" (1) to "more than two packs/day" (8) and alcohol: "If you drink alcohol, how much do you usually drink each time you drink," responses ranging from "I don't drink" (1) to "more than 6 drinks" (6).

Table 1 presents the psychosocial measures used in this study and their reliabilities. The psychometric properties of these scales have also been demonstrated in previous research (Botvin, Baker, Dusenbury, Tortu, and Botvin, 1990; Scheier and Botvin, 1995). Multi-item scales had reliabilities ranging from .52 for task persistence to .91 for ethnic identity.

Other measures not appropriate for inclusion in Table 1 assessed perceived social influence to use drugs, antisocial behavior, alcohol knowledge, marijuana knowledge, church attendance, self-reported absenteeism and grade point average. The social influence measures included perceived alcohol use by friends ("How many of your friends do you think drink alcohol"), perceived peer norms ("In your opinion, how many people your age drink alcoholic beverages"), perceived alcohol use ("how many adults do you think drink beer, wine, or liquor"), and perceived availability of alcohol use ("how easy is it to get beer, wine, or liquor"). Scales for the perceived drug use items ranged from "none" (1) to "all or almost all" (5) and for the availability item ranged from "very hard" (1) to "very easy" (6). Each social influence item was repeated for marijuana with the same stem and response format.

Self-reported grades were assessed on a five-point scale ranging from "D's or lower" (1) through "Mostly A's" (5). The measure of antisocial behavior consisted of three items tapping trouble at school, at home, or with the police and used a common stem for all three items ("How often in the past month did you get into trouble"). Responses ranged from "never" (1) through "more than four times" (5). The sum of these three responses was used as a relative index of delinquency. Church attendance was rated on an eight-point scale ranging from "never" (1) through "more than once a week" (8). School absenteeism was assessed on a five-point anchored scale ranging from "none" (1) through "16 or more days" (5).

TABLE 1. Reliabilities and Sources for Measures Used: Baseline Pretest Sample[1]

Psychosocial measure	Sample item	α	Principal source
Ethnic identity (5)	I have a lot of pride in my ethnic group and its accomplishments	.91	Phinney (1992)
Task persistence (4)	If something is really difficult, I get frustrated and quit	.52	Kendall & Wilcox (1979)
Sensation-seeking (6)	I enjoy fast driving	.74	Eysenck & Eysenck (1975)
Self-esteem (5)	I feel that I have a number of good qualities	.89	Rosenberg (1965)
Assertiveness (10)	How likely would you be to do the following things: Tell people your opinion, even if you know they will not agree with you	.82	Gambrill & Richey (1975)
Communication skills (4)	When I want to understand other people I: ask questions if they say something that isn't clear	.75	Botvin et al. (1994)
Decision-making skills (5)	Get the information needed to make the best choice	.90	Wills (1986)
Self-reinforcement (5)	I silently praise myself even for small achievements	.85	Heiby (1983)
Self-management (5)	If I feel sad, I try to think about pleasant things	.86	Rosenbaum (1980)
Anxiety symptoms (4)	I felt relaxed and free of tension	.59	Veit & Ware (1983) Langner (1962)

TABLE 1 (continued)

Psychosocial measure	Sample item	α	Principal source
Depressive symptoms (4)	*I felt downhearted or sad*	.55	Veit & Ware (1983)
Anxiety reduction skills (5)	*When I feel anxious, I: tell myself to feel calm and confident, and not worry*	.82	Botvin et al. (1994)
Bonding to school (5)	*Most mornings I look forward to going to school*	.79	Catalano et al. (1993)
Family management practices (5)	*My parents are stricter with me than most other parents*	.81	Catalano et al. (1993)
Drug refusal skills (5)	*If someone asked you to smoke, drink, use marijuana or other drugs: how likely would you: make up an excuse and leave*	.84	Botvin et al. (1996)
Drinking attitudes (5)	*Kids who drink have more friends*	.77	Botvin et al. (1990)

1 Sample restricted to minority youth (N = 4712). Numbers in parentheses reflect the number of items in the scale. Reliabilities were computed using Cronbach's alpha. Items scales range from: never (1) to always (5); strongly disagree (1) to strongly agree (5); definitely would (1) to definitely would not (5).
a Scales were either developed specifically for intervention program modules and have been tested in a five-year longitudinal study or were developed specifically for new program modules incorporated in current NIDA-funded study of multiethnic youth.

Four dichotomously scored ("true/false") items tapped knowledge of the prevalence of alcohol use (e.g., "most adults drink wine, beer, or liquor everyday") or the effects of alcohol (e.g., "drinking beer, wine, or liquor makes you more pepped up and alert") and were summed into a single scale. This procedure was repeated for knowledge items specific to marijuana and a separate scale was created.

Designation and Assignment of Risk/Protective Factors. Based on their respective distributions, a total of 32 individual measures were dichotomized using the upper (or respectively lower) 30th percentile. Past adolescent drug use research used cut-points ranging from the 20th-25th percentiles (e.g., Scheier and Newcomb, 1991). We used a more liberal 30th percentile, to widen the relative risk net that captures heightened or elevated vulnerability. To create binary risk factors, students in either the upper or lower 30th percentile depending on the scaling of the original measure, were assigned a "1" (designating them as "at-risk"), and the remaining portion of the distribution were assigned a "0" for no-risk. For example, distributions for the 4-item behavioral control item (assessing task persistence, attentiveness, and diligence) indicated that 33.2% of the sample at the pretest were considered being "at-risk," having low behavioral control scores. Guided by both Jessor's social-psychological model of problem behavior (Jessor and Jessor, 1977; Jessor, 1991) and developmental considerations, we assigned the 32 binary risk factors to one of nine additive risk indices. The nine additive indices included socioeconomic or background risk (nuclear living status, absenteeism, church attendance, and lunch status), social influence (perceived friends' alcohol use, perceived norms for peer and adult alcohol use, and perceived availability of alcohol), alcohol expectancies and knowledge, conventionality (antisocial behavior, sensation-seeking, family management, and school bonding), competence (self-reinforcement skills, self-management skills, decision-making skills, behavioral control [task persistence] and self-reported grades), affective distress (depressive and anxious symptomatology, self-esteem, and anxiety reduction skills), and social skills (assertiveness, communication skills, and drug-refusal skills). To avoid any confounding between alcohol- and marijuana-specific social influence items, a separate social influence risk index for marijuana containing measures related only to marijuana was created and likewise a cognitive-affective risk index containing scores for marijuana expectancies and marijuana knowledge was constructed, producing a total of nine risk indices at each assessment.

Data Analysis Approach

Several analytic strategies were employed to examine the role of psychosocial risk and alcohol and marijuana use. Analysis of variance procedures were used to examine mean levels of psychosocial risk and drug use by race and gender group (and included a race × gender interaction term). A second set of analyses examined the moderating influence of ethnic identity as it interacted with the risk indices in predicting both concurrent alcohol and marijuana use. Following the mediational logic proposed by Cohen and Cohen (1983) and subsequently elaborated by Baron and Kenny (1986), hierarchical multiple regression analyses were used, regressing the behavioral measures on the independent predictor(s), the moderator, and the interaction of these two terms. Significant moderation (i.e., buffering) is observed when the interaction term predicts unique variance in the outcome measure, controlling for the main effect terms. A third set of analyses utilized the longitudinal sample and, controlling for both early risk and initial alcohol (or separately marijuana) use, examined the relative predictive durability of the risk indices and the potential buffering effects of ethnic identity in accounting for general alcohol and marijuana involvement.

RESULTS

Subject Attrition

Prior to conducting longitudinal analyses of these data, analyses were conducted to determine if subject loss across the one-year follow-up period had any systematic effects on subsequent sample behavior(s). Overall, 28.2% of the pretest students were lost to attrition, despite aggressive tracking procedures. The slightly disproportionate representation of female students remained largely stable across time (53.5%), although there was a small but significantly larger loss of male students, $\chi^2(1) = 3.85, p < .05$. Dropouts were significantly more likely to report smoking marijuana, $\chi^2(1) = 26.32, p < .001$ and significantly more likely to smoke cigarettes $\chi^2(1) = 17.42, p < .001$. Attrition did not significantly affect loss of alcohol users.

In addition to conducting chi-square proportional analyses, mean comparisons indicated that dropouts reported higher levels of alcohol involvement (using a log transformed composite measure of frequency, intensity, and drunkenness), $t(851) = 2.33, p < .05$ and higher mean levels of marijuana use, $t(604) = 4.10, p < .001$. With respect to psychosocial risk, dropouts reported higher levels of social influence risk for both alcohol, $t(1797) = 2.61, p < .01$ and marijuana, $t(852) = 3.76, p < .001$. Dropouts also had lower competence, $t(826) = 3.66, p < .001$, less conventionality, $t(775) = 2.12, p < .05$, and more affective distress, $t(436) = 2.52, p < .05$. A regression model with stepwise inclusion indicated that only two risk indices significantly predicted retention status (dropouts coded as "0" and panel coded as "1"): social influences for marijuana use ($\beta = -.09, p < .01$) and personal competence ($\beta = -.12, p < .001$), and accounted for 2% of the variance. In summary, while there were a few significant differences in behavioral outcomes and psychosocial functioning between panel and dropout students, these differences accounted for relatively small amounts of variation in retention status.

Ethnic and Gender Differences in Drug Use Patterns

About one-third of the longitudinal sample reported some use of alcohol and 6.4% reported some use of marijuana at Time 1. Hispanic youth were more likely to have tried alcohol, $\chi^2(1) = 18.11, p < .001$, than African-American youth. Gender was not associated with drinking status. Likewise, race and gender were independent of self-reported marijuana use status. Hispanic youth reported significantly higher alcohol involvement, $t[1809] = 5.86, p < .001$.

A larger proportion of youth reported drinking (41%) and smoking marijuana (15.6%) at the end of 8th grade and there was a significant increase in the number of new drinkers (28.54%) and marijuana users (12.55%) from the seventh to the eighth grade (all p's $< .001$). Hispanic youth continued to report significantly higher mean levels of drinking ($t[1,1364] = 6.28, p < .001$), whereas African-American youth reported more marijuana use (Ms = 1.21 vs. 1.14, $t[1,1364] = 2.94, p < .01$). Males reported significantly more marijuana use (Ms = 1.22 vs. 1.13, $t[1,1364] = 3.21, p < .01$).

Ethnic and Gender Differences in Psychosocial Risk

Ethnic and gender differences in psychosocial risk were also examined using analysis of variance comparisons. Table 2 shows the results of these analyses both for students during the seventh grade and later during the eighth grade. At Time 1, in grade 7, African-Americans reported higher social influences to use marijuana than Hispanic youth, $t[1,1787] = 6.54, p < .001$; less competence $t[1,1799] = 4.81, p < .001$, and a significant ethnicity $\times$ gender interaction for affective distress (F$[1,933] = 6.41, p < .05$). Multiple range (post hoc) comparisons with Bonferroni adjustments indicated that African-American males reported the highest levels of distress, followed closely by Hispanic females, Hispanic males, and African-American females. Hispanic youth reported more sociodemographic risk ($t[1,1809] = 3.36, p < .001$).

TABLE 2. Risk Index Means by Race and Gender: Baseline (7th Grade) and One-Year Follow-Up (8th Grade)

Psychosocial Risk Index	Total Mean[a]	SD	African-American Male	African-American Female	Latino Male	Latino Female	Fisher's Exact Race[b]	Sex[b]	R × S
				Means (7th Grade)					
Alcohol Social Influences	1.32	1.16	1.99c	2.22	2.11	2.26			
Alcohol Cognitive-Affective	0.70	0.67	0.64	0.70	0.73	0.73			
Marijuana Social Influences	1.02	1.13	1.70	1.90	1.38	1.45	6.54***		
Marijuana Cognitive-Affective	0.48	0.61	0.47	0.49	0.49	0.44			
Conventionality	0.67	0.87	0.67	0.62	0.75	0.67			
Competence	0.69	0.98	0.65	0.55	0.83	0.83	4.81***		
Affective Distress	0.58	0.79	0.85	0.71	0.71	0.83			6.41***
Social Skills	0.76	0.76	0.80	0.76	0.77	0.68			
Sociodemographic	2.17	0.96	2.10	2.12	2.31	2.21	3.36***		
				Means (8th Grade)					
Alcohol Social Influences	1.30	1.22	1.07	1.29	1.36	1.57	4.30**		
Alcohol Cognitive-Affective	0.85	0.69	0.75	0.90	0.84	0.89		2.54*	
Marijuana Social Influences	1.55	1.33	1.63	1.77	1.21	1.43	4.94***	2.56*	
Marijuana Cognitive-Affective	0.77	0.69	0.68	0.86	0.67	0.81		4.03***	
Conventionality	0.99	1.05	0.88	0.89	1.21	1.04	4.04***		
Competence	1.02	1.11	1.00	0.89	1.27	1.07	3.73***	2.29*	
Affective Distress	0.78	0.95	0.71	0.72	0.84	0.89	2.64**		
Social Skills	0.85	0.78	0.90	0.88	0.80	0.75	2.49*		
Sociodemographic	1.67	0.97	1.66	1.60	1.74	1.75	2.05*		

a   Sample means unadjusted.
b   Main effects reported as t-values, significant interaction reported as F-value. Sample sizes vary because of missing data (Total sample N_1 = 938-1815; N_2 = 1087-1303).
c   Means for subgroups are least-squares. Alphas for post hoc comparisons adjusted to control for experiment-wise Type I error rate.

$^{\dagger}p < .10$, $^*p < .05$, $^{**}p < .01$, $^{***}p < .001$

At the end of the eighth grade, there were substantially more ethnic and gender differences in mean levels of psychosocial risk. Hispanic youth reported more alcohol-related social influence risk $t(1,1360) = 4.30$, $p < .001$, more unconventionality, $t(1,1309) = 4.04$, $p < .001$, more competence risk, $t(1,1363) = 3.73$, $p < .001$, more affective distress, $t(1,1131) = 2.64$, $p < .01$, and more sociodemographic risk, $t(1,1364) = 2.05$, $p < .05$. African-American youth, on the other hand, reported more social influences to use marijuana, $t(1,1360) = 4.93$, $p < .001$, and more social skills risk, $t(1,1269) = 2.48$, $p < .05$. There were also more significant gender differences at the end of the eighth grade than during the seventh grade. Females reported more perceived social influence risk for alcohol $(t[1,1360] = 3.20, p < .01)$ and marijuana $(t[1,1360] = 2.56, p < .05)$, more alcohol-related cognitive-affective risk $(t[1,1349] = 2.54$, $p < .05)$, more marijuana-related knowledge and more positive expectancies $(t[1,1348] = 4.03, p < .001)$, and males reported more competence risk $(t[1,1363] = 2.29, p < .05)$.

Ethnic Identity as a Moderator of Risk and Drug Use: Cross-Sectional Analyses

Utilizing the seventh grade cross-sectional data, we examined ethnic identity as a moderator of the effects of risk on drug use. Moderators operate in several ways including changing the direction of the relationship between the predictor and criterion or by lowering the magnitude of the association between the predictor and criterion. Moderation is demonstrated when the interaction between a moderator variable and predictor variable (represented as their cross-product term) adds significant unique variance when predicting the criterion (Cohen and Cohen, 1983). Although a variety of analytic techniques are available for detecting moderation, the most commonly used approach involves hierarchical moderated multiple regression with forced entry of predictor variables followed by inclusion of any interaction terms (Cohen and Cohen, 1983).

Table 3 contains the results of these analyses for both alcohol and marijuana use. Two out of the seven equations produced a significant interaction term for alcohol (cognitive-affective risk and social skills) and three significant interaction terms were obtained for marijuana (social influences, competence, and social skills). Using guidelines presented in Aiken and West (1991), the ethnic identity measure was trichotomized to reflect low (-1 SD), medium (centered on the mean), and high ($+1$ SD) levels of ethnic identity. Regression slopes for the equations containing significant interactions are plotted in Figure 1 for alcohol and Figure 2 for marijuana.

TABLE 3. Moderated Multiple Regression Statistics for Seventh Grade Cross-Sectional Data

Risk Domain	ΔR^2	F	β	SE
Corresponding Step		Alcohol[a]		
Cognitive-Affective	.033[b]	11.95***	.174***	.029
Ethnic Identity	.002	0.62	-.009	.005
CA × EI	.011	4.02*	.110*	.008
Social Skills	.002	0.85	.049	.024
Ethnic Identity	.003	0.96	.003	.005
SS × EI	.018	6.63*	-.146*	.006
Corresponding Step		Marijuana[c]		
Social Influences	.102	39.50***	.340	.011
Ethnic Identity	.006	2.41	-.059	.004
SI × EI	.010	4.04*	-.006	.003
Competence	.009	3.35†	.102†	.012
Ethnic Identity	.0001	0.04	-.091	.005
CP × EI	.012	4.20*	.137*	.003
Social Skills	.017	6.12*	.131	.017
Ethnic Identity	.002	0.07	-.002	.004
SS × EI	.011	3.86*	-.112*	.004

a   A composite measure of frequency, intensity, and drunkenness, natural logarithm transformed plus 1.
b   Initial step is zero-order bivariate correlation. Subsequent steps reflect incremental R^2, significance level corresponds to incremental R^2 and corresponding F-change.
c   A composite measure of frequency and intensity, natural logarithm transformed plus 1.

†$p < .10$, *$p < .05$, **$p < .01$, ***$p < .001$

As depicted, the graphs for alcohol represent disordinal interactions, where the rank ordering of the ethnic identity groups changes as risk increases. The plot of alcohol use by cognitive-affective risk status (Figure 1a) shows that the high ethnic identity group is at greatest risk for alcohol involvement, whereas the low ethnic identity group is at lower risk for alcohol involvement. Figure 1b shows that youth who have low ethnic identity and high social skills risk are at greatest risk for alcohol use, whereas youth reporting low ethnic identity and low social skills risk are at lowest risk for alcohol use.

The graphs (Figures 2a, b, c) depicting the findings of the moderation analyses with marijuana use confirm our hypotheses regarding the buffer-

FIGURE 1. Plot of the Significant Buffering Effects of Ethnic Identity: Log-Transformed Alcohol Use

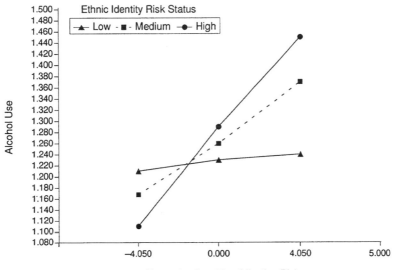

Figure 1a. Cognitive-Affective Risk

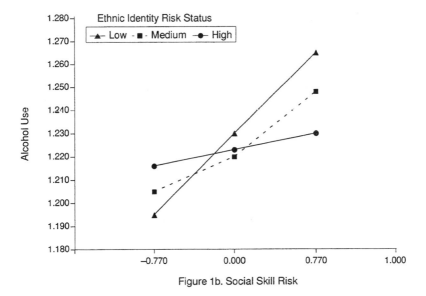

Figure 1b. Social Skill Risk

FIGURE 2. Plot of the Significant Buffering Effects of Ethnic Identity: Log-Transformed Marijuana Use

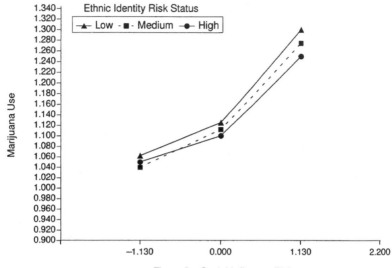

Figure 2a. Social Influence Risk

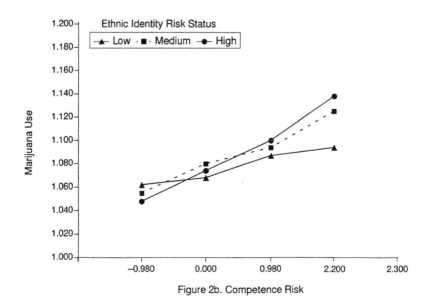

Figure 2b. Competence Risk

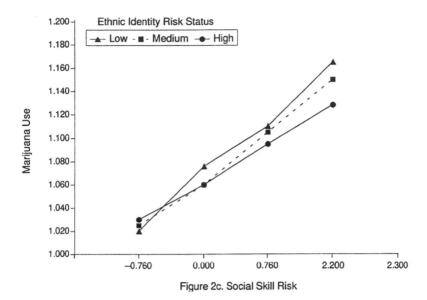

Figure 2c. Social Skill Risk

ing effects of ethnic identity. With respect to social influence risk, there is a partial crossover effect for ethnic identity. The rank position of the high ethnic identity group changes as social influence risk increases. The low ethnic identity group remains at highest risk for marijuana use and this remains so, irrespective of social influence risk status. Figure 2b also demonstrates the crossover effect with the high ethnic identity group at lowest risk for marijuana use and at low levels of competence risk, whereas at higher levels of competence risk, the high ethnic identity group is at the highest risk for marijuana use. The model containing social skills risk (Figure 2c) also contains a crossover effect and shows a protective effect at high levels of ethnic identity and social skills risk.

To determine if the individual interaction terms maintain their predictive significance when specified with other types of risk, we also tested a model that included all seven risk indices and the two significant interaction terms for alcohol. This model was repeated for the three significant interaction terms obtained for marijuana including the marijuana-specific risk indices. In the model containing alcohol as the criterion, the seven risk indices were entered blockwise, followed hierarchically by ethnic identity and the two significant interaction terms. In the final step, the skills $\times$ ethnic identity term was significant ($\beta = -.12, p < .05$) and the cognitive-affective risk $\times$ ethnic identity term approaches significance ($\beta = .08, p < .10$). The incremental R^2 and the corresponding F-value for the final step were significant ($\Delta R^2 = 2.1\%$, $F = 9.55$, $p < .01$). For marijuana use, on the other hand, both the competence and skills interaction terms remained significant, controlling for all other levels of risk: competence × ethnic identity ($\beta = .13$, $p < .05$) and social skills ($\beta = -.11$, $p < .05$) ($\Delta R^2 = 2.2\%$, $F = 9.40$, $p < .01$).

Ethnic Identity as a Moderator of Risk and Drug Use: Longitudinal Analyses

The longitudinal models also utilized moderated multiple regression techniques using eighth grade behavioral measures as the criterion and controlling for seventh grade levels of alcohol or marijuana use, respectively, and seventh grade levels of psychosocial risk. Again, separate regression models were conducted for each risk index with the specified order of entry hierarchically including the covariates (seventh grade use and psychosocial risk), eighth grade psychosocial risk and ethnic identity,[1] and the cross multiplication of these terms.

The results of the longitudinal regression analyses are contained in Table 4. Only one of the seven equations produced a significant interaction term and this involved social skills risk and alcohol use. The full model accounted for 20% of the variance in drinking, $F(5,645) = 32.72$, $p < .001$, and the partial effect associated with the interaction term contributed slightly under 1% to the model variation, $F = 6.79$, $p < .01$. Significant regression parameters at the final step included seventh grade alcohol use ($\beta = .39$, $p < .001$), eighth grade social skills risk ($\beta = .16$, $p < .001$), and the interaction term ($\beta = .095$, $p < .01$). There were no significant interaction terms for the marijuana analyses, although there was a marginal trend for affective distress ($\beta = -.09$, $p < .10$, $F = 3.52$).

We also ran an empirically reduced model that included only those seventh grade and eighth grade risk indices that accounted for significant portions of variation in the criterion and included the social skills × ethnic identity interaction term. This model tests whether the interaction remains significant controlling for all other levels of risk during both the seventh and eighth grades. A fully saturated model including seventh grade drinking, all of the seventh grade and eighth grade risk indices, ethnic identity, and an interaction term (ethnic identity × social skills risk) accounted for 37% of the variance in drinking behavior, $F(16, 467) = 16.10$, $p < .0001$. The skills × ethnic identity interaction term was marginally significant ($\beta = .07$, $p < .10$). Significant predictors in this model also included seventh grade drinking ($\beta = .26$, $p < .001$), seventh grade social influence risk ($\beta = -.10$, $p < .05$), eighth grade social influence risk ($\beta = .32$, $p < .001$), eighth grade conventionality risk (lowered family management skills,

TABLE 4. Moderated Multiple Regression Statistics for Longitudinal Data

Eighth Grade	Alcohol Model Statistics[a]				Marijuana Model Statistics			
Risk Domain	ΔR^2	F	β	SE	ΔR^2	F	β	SE
Social Influences (SI)	.28	95.23***	.368***	.014	.26	88.36***	.33***	.012
Ethnic Identity (EI)	.003	3.20[m]	.056[m]	.004	.001	0.54	−.020	.004
SI × EI	---[b]	---	---	---	.001	0.79	−.029	.003
Cognitive-Affective (CA)	.16	45.66***	−.062[m]	.004	.14	37.25***	−.090*	.023
Ethnic Identity (EI)	.003	2.73[m]	.063[m]	.004	.001	0.69	−.024	.004
CA × EI	.001	1.12	−.040	.006	.0015	1.19	.040	.005
Conventionality (CV)	.25	79.06***	.287***	.015	.17	45.67***	.212***	.015
Ethnic Identity (EI)	.004	3.71[m]	.053	.004	---[b]	---	.006	.004
CV × EI	.001	0.75	.030	.003	.0015	1.19	−.040	.003
Competence (CP)	.16	48.24***	.089***	.017	.14	37.29***	.084*	.014
Ethnic Identity (EI)	.008	6.72**	.091**	.004	---	---	.017	.004
CP × EI	---	---	---	---	.003	2.60	−.061	.003
Social Skills (SS)	.19	51.15***	.160***	.022	.16	41.13***	.219***	.019
Ethnic Identity (EI)	.002	1.75	.021	.004	.001	0.71	−.043	.004
SS × EI	.008	6.79**	.095**	.005	.002	1.40	.045	.005
Affective Distress (AD)	.15	29.64***	.165***	.021	.09	17.00***	.050	.019
Ethnic Identity (EI)	.005	3.11[m]	.077[m]	.006	---	---	.045	.005
AD × EI	---	---	---	---	.007	3.52[m]	−.091[m]	.004
Sociodemographic (SD)	.15	44.23	.048	.019	.13	36.27***	.080*	.018
Ethnic Identity (EI)	.004	3.84[m]	.064[m]	.004	.001	0.58	−.030	.004
SD × EI	.0015	1.34	.039	.004	---	---	---	---

[a] Model fit statistics include controls for Time 1 consumption and Time 1 risk. R^2 at initial step corresponds to model plus covariates whereas successive R^2's are incremental variance (partial regression coefficient). β's reflect standardized regression parameters at final step.
[b] Parameter not estimated ($p > .05$ F-to-enter).
*$p < .05$, **$p < .01$, ***$p < .001$, [m]$p < .10$

lowered school bonding, deviant behavior, and high sensation seeking: β = .21, $p <$ .001), eighth grade social skills risk (β = .11, $p <$ .01), and eighth grade affective distress risk (β = .08, $p <$ .05). In a second step, the nonsignificant predictors were eliminated from the saturated model and a final model was obtained that included seventh grade drinking (β = .26, $p <$ .001), seventh grade conventionality risk (β = .07, $p <$ .10), eighth grade social influence risk (β = .30, $p <$ .05), eighth grade conventionality (β = .22, $p <$ .001), eighth grade social skills risk (β = .09, $p <$ .01), and the interaction of social skills risk and ethnic identity (β = .06, $p <$ .10). The reduced model accounted for 36% of the variance in drinking behavior, F (7, 703) = 56.26, $p <$ .001, indicating that there was little degradation in the fit of this model compared to the saturated model with all seventh and eighth grade risk indices.

DISCUSSION

This study examined the role of ethnic identity as a moderator of the relationship between several distinct classes of psychosocial risk for alcohol and marijuana use, both concurrently and longitudinally in a cohort of minority youth. Early adolescence is a time when many youth first experiment with alcohol and other drugs. It is also during this period that youth actively begin to form a more coherent sense of identity. In addition to the major developmental tasks that are the hallmark of this period for all adolescents, minority youth must also deal with issues of ethnic self-identification and ethnic validation and the integration of their ethnic and personal identity. Because of the relative salience of these tasks, it is an ideal time to examine the role of identity processes in the development of alcohol and drug use behavior. It was hypothesized that ethnic factors would play a major role in determining vulnerability to alcohol and marijuana drug use. Specifically, it was posited that high ethnic identity would offset either social influences or intrapersonal motivations to drink alcohol or use marijuana.

The sample of youth we examined reported levels of alcohol and marijuana use consistent with recently obtained national estimates for a similar age group. Overall, one-third of these youth reported some use of alcohol in the seventh grade, and by the eighth grade this proportion had significantly increased to 41%. Marijuana use was reported by 6.4% of the seventh graders and increased to 15.6% by the eighth grade. Recent data from the National Household Survey on Drug Abuse (NHSDA, 1995) found that 41.7% of 12-15 year olds used alcohol and 14.4% used marijuana.

The impact of ethnic identity on drug use was highlighted by the results of both cross-sectional and longitudinal data. However, most of the significant interactions were obtained using the cross-sectional data. The pattern and form of the interactions revealed essentially two distinct processes by which ethnic identity influences the relationship between psychosocial risk and drug use. Low levels of ethnic identity were associated with both low risk and low use; at higher levels of risk, low ethnic identity was associated with high levels of drug use. This finding is consistent with a stress-buffering interpretation and indicates that high identity offsets or diminishes the negative effect of risk.

In two instances, however, high levels of ethnic identity were associated with high levels of risk and drug use. These findings were specific to competence risk and marijuana use, and cognitive-affective risk and alcohol use. With respect to cognitive-affective risk (low knowledge and positive drug use expectancies), the functional role of deviant peer bonding may offer a viable explanation for the finding that the role of ethnic identity was the opposite of what was hypothesized, suggesting that social influences play a large role in promoting drug use irrespective of the nature or origins of these social influences. Youth low in competence (at high risk) may attempt to offset feelings of distress and self-derogation by bonding with deviant peers. A by-product of bonding to a deviant or unconventional peer group is that it may provide a means of obtaining information about drugs and their effects, two important components in the decision to use drugs (Scheier and Botvin, 1997).

The findings from the longitudinal analyses provide further evidence that ethnic factors may emerge over time and play an independent role in the initiation of drug use. When controlling for seventh grade drinking, and eighth grade risk, ethnic identity significantly and uniquely predicted alcohol use in a model including competence risk. There was also a trend for unique effects in the models containing social influence risk, cognitive-affective risk, conventionality, affective distress, and sociodemographic risk. In addition to these findings, the measures of risk included in this study were found to be substantial and significant predictors of concurrent alcohol and marijuana use. Over time, these determinants gained in explanatory power, accounting for larger portions of variance during the eighth grade than in the seventh grade. The findings from the longitudinal analyses also indicate that, controlling for early levels of risk, ethnic factors still accounted for significant portions of variance in alcohol use.

Notwithstanding the importance of these findings, there are several limitations to this study. First, the small sample size for some of the cross-sectional moderator analyses (limited by the low response rate to the ethnic identity items) may have hampered our ability to detect significance. The ethnic identity items were located toward the end of the survey and fatigue may have contributed to the lower completion rate for these items. Second, the measure of ethnic identity was based on four items that represented only one aspect of ethnic identity. Phinney (1992) and others have encouraged the use of much longer measures to assess the full spectrum of ethnic identity. Thus, the absence of stronger evidence for the moderator effect of ethnic identity in the longitudinal analyses may be the result of measurement limitations. Future studies should replicate these findings with a more comprehensive measure of ethnic identity.

Third, several factors typically contribute to difficulty in detecting significant moderator effects (McClelland and Judd, 1993). Variability of the joint term (and heteroscedasticity of the residual), the form or shape of the distribution of the interaction term, and the strength of the association among the variables entered into the model often determine the statistical power of the test for significance of the interaction. The sum total of these statistical problems is a failure to control Type II error, which leads to the erroneous acceptance of a false null hypothesis. Despite our efforts to control for many of these potential confounds, future studies should address these issues with greater precision. By their very nature, moderator variables and the operation of interactions are complex and often difficult to interpret. However, attempts to unravel these relationships are important to further our understanding of the role of risk factors in drug use among minority youth.

Finally, this study was conducted entirely within an exploratory framework. A complete understanding of the mechanisms of action for ethnic identity and drug use are still in the preliminary stages of discovery. Necessarily, only a limited set of variables associated with drug use and ethnic identity was included in this study. Future studies should include a broader range of risk factors in order to increase our understanding of how ethnic identity and other cultural factors interact with interpersonal and intrapersonal risk factors. However, despite the limitations of this study, these findings provide important new information about the role of ethnic identity and the initiation of drug use that may help refine current prevention approaches and increase their effectiveness with minority youth.

ENDNOTE

1. Ethnic identity assessed in the eighth grade was used because the seventh grade measure had a large amount of missing data. The ethnic identity questions appeared at the end of the survey, and in the seventh grade assessment, reading

comprehension and fatigue may have limited the response rates for these items (and any items appearing subsequent in the survey). A full year and grade level later, almost twice the number of students responded to these items. We also felt that using the eighth grade measure of ethnic identity would be more conceptually appropriate, particularly because Cross (1985) and others (Knight et al., 1993) have argued that this age represents a critical juncture point for initiating the developmental process of ethnic identity consolidation. Therefore, we postulated that the use of the Time 3 measure would introduce more meaningful variance.

REFERENCES

Aboud, F. E. (1987). The development of ethnic self-identification and attitudes. In J. S. Phinney & M. J. Rotheram (Eds.), *Childrens' ethnic socialization* (pp. 32-55). Newbury Park, CA: Sage Publications.

Aiken, L. S., & West, S. G. (1991). *Multiple regression: Testing and interpreting interactions.* Newbury Park, CA: Sage.

Arroyo, C. G., & Zigler, E. (1995). Racial identity, academic achievement, and the psychological well-being of economically disadvantaged adolescents. *Journal of Personality and Social Psychology, 69,* 903-914.

Bachman, J. G., Wallace, J. M., O'Malley, P. M., Johnston, L. D., Kurth, C. L., & Neighbors, H. W. (1991). Racial/ethnic differences in smoking, drinking, and illicit drug use among American high school seniors, 1976-89. *American Journal of Public Health, 81,* 372-377.

Barnes, G. M., & Welte, J. W. (1986). Adolescent alcohol abuse: Subgroup differences and relationships to other problem behaviors. *Journal of Adolescent Research, 1,* 79-94.

Baron, R. M., & Kenny, D. A. (1986). The moderator-mediator variable distinction in social psychological research: Conceptual, strategic, and statistical considerations. *Journal of Personality and Social Psychology, 51,* 1173-1182.

Bautista de Domanico, Y., Crawford, I., & De Wolfe, A. S. (1994). Ethnic identity and self-concept in Mexican-American adolescents: Is bicultural identity related to stress or better adjustment? *Child and Youth Care Forum, 23,* 197-206.

Bernal, M. E., Saenz, D. S., & Knight, G. P. (1991). Ethnic identity and adaptation of Mexican American youths in school settings. *Hispanic Journal of the Behavioral Sciences, 13,* 135-154.

Botvin, G. J., Baker, E., Dusenbury, L., Tortu, S., & Botvin, E. M. (1990). Preventing adolescent drug abuse through a multimodal cognitive-behavioral approach: Results of a 3-year study. *Journal of Consulting and Clinical Psychology, 58,* 437-446.

Botvin, G. J., Schinke, S. P., Epstein, J. A., & Diaz, T. (1994). Effectiveness of culturally-focused and generic skills training approaches to alcohol and drug abuse prevention among minority youths. *Psychology of Addictive Behaviors, 8,* 116-127.

Botvin, G. J., Schinke, S., & Orlandi, M. A. (1996). Interim Center Project Report to the National Institute on Drug Abuse (P50DA7656–Center for the Study of Multiethnic Drug Abuse).

Bry, B. H. (1983). Predicting drug abuse: Review and reformulation. *The International Journal of the Addictions, 18*, 223-233.

Bry, B. H., McKeon, P., & Pandina, R. J. (1982). Extent of drug use as a function of number of risk factors. *Journal of Abnormal Psychology, 91*, 273-279.

Catalano, R. F., Hawkins, J. D., Krenz, C., Gillmore, M., Morrison, D., Wells, E., & Abbott, R. (1993). Using research to guide culturally appropriate drug abuse prevention. *Journal of Consulting and Clinical Psychology, 61*, 804-811.

Cohen, J., & Cohen, P. (1983). *Applied multiple regression/correlation analysis for the behavioral sciences* (2nd ed.). Hillsdale, NJ: Erlbaum.

Cohen, S., & Wills, T. A. (1985). Stress, social support, and the buffering hypothesis. *Psychological Bulletin, 98*, 310-357.

Collins, R. L. (1995). Issues of ethnicity in research on the prevention of substance abuse. In G. J. Botvin, S. Schinke, & M. A. Orlandi (Eds.), *Drug Abuse Prevention with Multiethnic Youth*. Thousand Oaks, CA: Sage Publications.

Cross, W. E. (1985). Black identity: Rediscovering the distinction between personal identity and reference group orientation. In M. B. Spencer, G. K. Brookins, & W. R. Allen (Eds.), *Beginnings: The social and affective development of black children* (pp. 155-171). Hillsdale, NJ: Erlbaum.

Dembo, R., Allen, N., Farrow, D., Schmeidler, J., & Burgos, W. (1985). A causal analysis of early drug involvement in three inner-city neighborhood settings. *The International Journal of the Addictions, 20*, 1213-1237.

Dembo, R., Burgos, W., Des Jarlais, D., & Schmeidler, L. (1979). Ethnicity and drug use among urban high school youths. *The International Journal of the Addictions, 14*, 557-568.

Erikson, E. H. (1968). *Identity: Youth and crisis*. New York: W. W. Norton.

Eysenck, H. J., & Eysenck, S. B. G. (1975). *Manual of the Eysenck personality questionnaire*. London: Hodder & Stoughton.

Farrell, A. D., Danish, S. J., & Howard, C. W. (1992). Relationship between drug use and other problem behaviors in urban adolescents. *Journal of Consulting and Clinical Psychology, 60*, 705-712.

Felix-Ortiz, M., & Newcomb, M. D. (1995). Cultural identity and drug use among Latino and Latina adolescents. In G. J. Botvin, S. Schinke, & M. A. Orlandi (Eds.), *Drug Abuse Prevention with Multiethnic Youth* (pp. 147-165). Newbury Park, CA: Sage Publications.

Flannery, D. J., Vazsonyi, A. T., Torquati, J., & Fridrich, A. (1994). Ethnic and gender differences in risk for early adolescent substance use. *Journal of Youth and Adolescence, 23*, 195-213.

Gambrill, E. D., & Richey, C. A. (1975). An assertion inventory for use in assessment and research. *Behavior Therapy, 6*, 550-561.

Hawkins, J. D., Catalano, R. F., & Miller, J. Y. (1992). Risk and protective factors for alcohol and other drug problems in adolescence and early adulthood: Implications for substance abuse prevention. *Psychological Bulletin, 112*, 64-105.

Heiby, E. M. (1983). Assessment of frequency of self-reinforcement. *Journal of Personality and Social Psychology, 44,* 1304-1307.

Jessor, R. (1991). Risk behavior in adolescence: A psychosocial framework for understanding and action. *Journal of Adolescent Health, 12,* 597-605.

Jessor, R., & Jessor, S. L. (1977). *Problem behavior and psychosocial development: A longitudinal study of youth.* New York: Academic Press.

Johnston, L. D., O'Malley, P. M., & Bachman, J. G. (1995). *National Survey Results on Drug Use from the Monitoring the Future Study, 1975-1994. Vol. I Secondary School Students.* Washington, DC: U.S. Department of Health and Human Services. (NIH Publication No. 95-4026).

Kendall, P. C., & Wilcox, L. E. (1979). Self-control in children: Development of a rating scale. *Journal of Consulting and Clinical Psychology, 47,* 1020-1029.

Knight, G. P., Cota, M. K., & Bernal, M. E. (1993). The socialization of cooperative, competitive, and individualistic preferences among Mexican American children: The mediating role of ethnic identity. *Hispanic Journal of Behavioral Science, 15,* 291-309.

Langner, T. S. (1962). A twenty-two item screening score of psychiatric symptoms indicating impairment. *Journal of Health and Human Behavior, 3,* 269-276.

Maddahian, E., Newcomb, M. D., & Bentler, P. M. (1985). Single and multiple patterns of adolescent substance use: Longitudinal comparisons of four ethnic groups. *Journal of Drug Education, 15,* 311-326.

Maddahian, E., Newcomb, M. D., & Bentler, P. M. (1988). Risk factors for substance use: Ethnic differences among adolescents. *Journal of Substance Abuse, 1,* 11-23.

McClelland, G. H., & Judd, C. M. (1993). Statistical difficulties of detecting interactions and moderator effects. *Psychological Bulletin, 114,* 376-390.

Montgomery, G. T. (1992). Acculturation, stressors, and somatization patterns among students from extreme South Texas. *Hispanic Journal of Behavioral Sciences, 14,* 434-454.

Newcomb, M. D. (1992). Understanding the multidimensional nature of drug use and abuse: The role of consumption, risk factors, and protective factors. In M. Glantz & R. Pickens (Eds.), *Vulnerability to drug abuse* (pp. 255-297). Washington, DC: American Psychological Association.

Newcomb, M. D., Maddahian, E., & Bentler, P. M. (1986). Risk factors for drug use among adolescents: Concurrent and longitudinal analyses. *American Journal of Public Health, 76*(5), 525-531.

NHSDA (1995). *National Household Survey on Drug Abuse: Population Estimates, 1994* (DHHS Publication No. SMA 95-3063). Rockville, MD: Substance Abuse and Mental Health Services Administration.

Pearlin, L. I., Menaghan, E. G., Lieberman, M. A., & Mullan, J. T. (1981). The stress process. *Journal of Health and Social Behavior, 22,* 337-356.

Petraitis, J., Flay, B. R., & Miller, T. Q. (1995). Reviewing theories of adolescent substance use: Organizing pieces in the puzzle. *Psychological Bulletin, 117,* 67-86.

Phinney, J. S. (1989). Stages of ethnic identity development in minority group adolescents. *Journal of Early Adolescence, 9*, 34-49.

Phinney, J. S. (1990). Ethnic identity in adolescents and adults: Review of research. *Psychological Bulletin, 108*, 499-514.

Phinney, J. S. (1992). The multi-group ethnic identity measure: A new scale for use with diverse groups. *Journal of Adolescent Research, 7*, 156-176.

Phinney, J. S. (1993). Ethnic identity development in adolescence. In M. E. Bernal & G. P. Knight (Eds.), *Ethnic identity: Formation and transmission among Hispanics and other minorities* (pp. 61-79). Albany, NY: State University of New York Press.

Phinney, J. S., Lochner, B., & Murphy, R. (1990). Ethnic identity development and psychological adjustment in adolescence. In A. Stiffman & L. Davis (Eds.), *Advances in adolescent mental health, Vol V: Ethnic issues* (pp. 53-72). Newbury Park, CA: Sage.

Pooling Project Research Group (1978). Relationship of blood pressure, serum cholesterol, smoking habit, relative weight, and ECG abnormalities to incidence of major coronary events: Final report of the Pooling Project [Special Issue]. *Journal of Chronic Diseases, 31*, 201-306.

Rosenbaum, M. (1980). Schedule for assessing self-control behaviors. *Behavior Therapy, 11*, 109-121.

Rosenberg, M. (1965). *Society and the adolescent self-image.* Princeton: Princeton University Press.

Scheier, L. M., & Botvin, G. J. (1995). Effects of early adolescent drug use on cognitive efficacy in early-late adolescence: A developmental structural model. *Journal of Substance Abuse, 7*, 379-404.

Scheier, L. M., & Botvin, G. J. (1997). Expectancies as mediators of the effects of social influences and alcohol knowledge on adolescent alcohol use: A prospective analysis. *Psychology of Addictive Behaviors.*

Scheier, L. M., & Newcomb, M. D. (1991). Psychosocial predictors of drug use initiation and escalation: An expansion of the multiple risk factors hypothesis using longitudinal data. *Contemporary Drug Problems, 18*, 31-73.

Spencer, M. B. (1985). Cultural cognition and social cognition as identity correlates of Black children's personal-social development. In M. B. Spencer, G. K. Brookins, & W. R. Allen (Eds.), *Beginnings: The social and affective development of Black children* (pp. 215-230). Hillsdale, NJ: Lawrence Erlbaum.

Trimble, J. E. (1995). Toward an understanding of ethnicity and ethnic identity, and their relationship with drug use research. In G. J. Botvin, S. Schinke, & M. A. Orlandi (Eds.), *Drug Abuse Prevention with Multiethnic Youth* (pp. 3-27). Thousand Oaks, CA: Sage.

United States Bureau of the Census (1992). Population projections of the United States, by age, sex, race, and Hispanic origin: 1992 to 2050. *Current Population Reports*, Series P25-1092. Washington, DC: U.S. Government Printing Office.

Veit, C. T., & Ware, J. E. (1983). The structure of psychological distress and well-being in general populations. *Journal of Consulting and Clinical Psychology*, *51*, 730-742.

Whaley, A. L. (1993). Self-esteem, cultural identity, and psychosocial adjustment in African American children. *Journal of Black Psychology*, *19*, 406-422.

Wills, T. A. (1986). Stress and coping in early adolescence: Relationships to substance use in urban school samples. *Health Psychology*, *5*(6), 503-529.

Developing and Implementing Interventions in Community Settings

Steven Schinke
Kristin Cole
Tracy Diaz
Gilbert J. Botvin

SUMMARY. This paper describes the needs of youth at high risk of future drug use and an intervention approach which responds to those needs by utilizing community settings. The paper begins by discussing the merits of community-based drug abuse prevention. Next, the paper reviews the background and nature of drug use among youth who are at inordinately high risk for using and encountering problems associated with drugs. Against that backdrop, the authors offer an approach to intervening with high-risk youth to prevent drug use and its attendant problems. The community-based preventive intervention approach includes relevant theory, applicable principles and specific strategies. Results from community-based prevention interventions are next discussed. Finally, the authors summarize the strengths and limitations of a community-based prevention approach

Steven Schinke, PhD, and Kristin Cole, MA, are affiliated with Columbia University School of Social Work, 622 West 113th Street, New York, NY 10025. Tracy Diaz, MA, and Gilbert J. Botvin, PhD, are affiliated with the Institute for Prevention Research, Cornell University Medical College, 411 East 69th Street, New York, NY 10021.

Research reported in this paper was supported in part by the National Institute on Drug Abuse (DA05321).

[Haworth co-indexing entry note]: "Developing and Implementing Interventions in Community Settings." Schinke, Steven et al. Co-published simultaneously in *Journal of Child & Adolescent Substance Abuse* (The Haworth Press, Inc.) Vol. 6, No. 1, 1997, pp. 49-67; and: *The Etiology and Prevention of Drug Abuse Among Minority Youth* (ed: Gilbert J. Botvin, and Steven Schinke) The Haworth Press, Inc., 1997, pp. 49-67. Single or multiple copies of this article are available for a fee from The Haworth Document Delivery Service [1-800-342-9678, 9:00 a.m. - 5:00 p.m. (EST). E-mail address: getinfo@haworth.com].

49

offered to combat problems of drug use among high-risk youth. *[Article copies available for a fee from The Haworth Document Delivery Service: 1-800-342-9678. E-mail address: getinfo@haworth.com]*

KEYWORDS. Drug Use, Community-Based, Prevention, Adolescent

Intervening with youths, who are at risk for drug use, in their communities rather than through the school system, has several advantages. Frequently, researchers have trouble persuading school administrators and teachers to release class time for an intervention. Working with community centers avoids this problem since the nonschool day is longer than the school day. Community centers also operate on weekends, thereby creating additional opportunities for intervention hours. Thus, scheduling interventions in community centers is easier than in traditional school-based programs.

Another important advantage is that children in community centers choose to be there, rather than their mandated attendance at school. The community center is typically perceived as a more neutral ground than is the school for many at-risk youth. What is more, youth who do not perform well in school may be disinclined to participate in an intervention that is delivered at school. Similarly, at-risk youths frequently have parents that had negative experiences with schools, thus making them averse to school-based efforts. The community center is free of such prejudices.

Implementing drug abuse prevention in the community makes sense because substance experimentation usually takes place outside of school and in the community. Community centers have access to a more varied age group of youths. Furthermore, many of the youths most at risk for drug use do not attend school regularly or drop out altogether.

For researchers, using the community center as the unit of analysis, as opposed to a school, eases the research process because participating community centers do not have to be comparably sized. Small community agencies serve research purposes just as well as large community agencies. On the other hand, contamination is a greater concern. Intervention delivery in the community is vulnerable to overlap with other intervention efforts as youths in the community center may attend a variety of other programs or schools.

BACKGROUND

The primary prevention of risk-taking behavior among high-risk children and adolescents in this country continues to challenge practitioners, scientists, and policy makers. Particularly refractory to preventive intervention efforts are risk-taking problems of alcohol and other drug use. According to the National Institute on Drug Abuse, America's youth are the largest consumers of illicit drugs in the industrialized nations of the world (National Institute on Drug Abuse, 1985). After a decade-long downward trend in drug use, recent national survey data (Johnston, O'Malley and Bachman, 1995) show sharp increases in drug use among American adolescents.

Adolescents from ethnic-racial minority groups are at particularly high risk for drug use (Schinke, Bebel, Orlandi and Botvin, 1988). Tobacco, alcohol, and other drug use is also prevalent among economically disadvantaged Americans (Pavkov, McGovern and Geffner, 1993; Walter, Vaughan and Cohall, 1991). Behavioral patterns associated with increased drug use are more common among young people from households with incomes below the poverty line than among youth from less impoverished households (Dusenbury et al., 1992; Hechinger, 1992; Hiatt, Klatsky and Armstrong, 1988; Walter et al., 1992). Compared with their economically advantaged counterparts, poor people use substances earlier, heavier, and more habitually (U. S. Department of Health and Human Services, 1990).

For many youth, minority status is associated with low socioeconomic status (U. S. Congress Office of Technology Assessment, 1991; U. S. Congress Office of Technology Assessment, 1986). One study found that about 45 percent of all African-American children live in female-headed households. Of these children, 70 percent are poor (Center for the Study of Social Policy, 1986). To be sure, minority status does not necessarily equate with socioeconomic disadvantage, but institutional racism and other insidious forces place these youth at greater risk than majority culture youth for a host of problems. Once addicted or accustomed to drug use, African-American and Hispanic youth are less apt than their majority culture counterparts to stop smoking, reduce their drinking, or quit using drugs (Institute of Medicine, 1991; National Substance Abuse Institute, 1991). Although innovative approaches to preventing drug abuse have emerged in recent years, new intervention approaches are needed for these vulnerable youth (Bambade and Chalmers, 1991; Goplerud, 1991; Johnson, 1990; Schinke, Orlandi and Cole, 1992).

PREVENTION APPROACHES

Recent years have witnessed considerable research demonstrating that skills-based prevention interventions offer a promising approach to drug abuse problems among youth (Botvin and Wills, 1985; Flay, 1985; Fraser and Kohlert, 1988). Especially promising are interventions that focus on enhancing personal and social skills using cognitive-behavioral problem solving, decision making, and communication elements (Pentz, 1983; Schinke and Gilchrist, 1984).

Despite the promise of skills interventions, community-based approaches to prevent drug abuse among youth at highest risk for habitual and damaging use patterns are still lacking (Department of Health and Human Services, 1985; Fraser and Kohlert, 1988; Greenwald, Cullen and McKenna, 1987; McKay, Murphy, McGuire, Rivinus and Maisto, 1992; Zigler, Taussig and Black, 1992). Among the reasons for the limited testing of such approaches for community settings are research designs that favor studies with stable, compliant, homogeneous populations. School-based studies, the venue for most skills intervention research, are apt to overlook high-risk ethnic-racial minority group youth. Investigations are further hampered by limited access to ethnic-community institutions and by the lack of viable collaborations between research groups and community agencies and institutions.

PREVENTION FOR COMMUNITY SETTINGS

Implementing community-based interventions can potentially overcome the traditional impediments faced by drug abuse researchers. Targeting youth served by community-based agencies can reach those youth who are at highest risk for drug abuse and other problems and who are sorely in need of responsive preventive intervention services. An illustrative prevention approach for working with high-risk youths in community settings is presented in the following section. This approach draws on relevant theory as well as the authors' past work with skills interventions, high-risk youth, and preventive interventions.

Theory

Theories on the etiology of risk taking during adolescence have value for directing drug abuse prevention strategies. Rather than defining risk taking as pathological, early theorists viewed youthful deviance as resulting from socially induced pressures and normal developmental needs to achieve socially desirable goals (Cloward and Ohlin, 1960). Later, theorists perceived drug use and other risk taking among youth as a result of weak ties to conventional norms (Hirschi, 1969). Building on these tenets, subsequent theorists saw a pattern of risk taking as occurring when youths' conventional social bonds are neutralized through attenuating experiences (Elliot, Ageton and Canter, 1979). Recently, four theories have emerged to further explain risk taking in adolescence and to guide strategies aimed at preventing drug use among high-risk youth in community settings. These theories are social learning theory, problem behavior theory, peer cluster theory, and family networks theory.

Social Learning Theory. According to social learning theory, people learn how to behave through a process of modeling and reinforcement (Bandura, 1977). Moreover, according to this theory, youths' perceptions that deviant behaviors are standard practice among their peers may promote deviance through the establishment of negative normative beliefs. Such perceptions may tell adolescents that deviant acts are socially acceptable and that these acts are necessary to be popular, grown up, and sophisticated. Perceived payoffs for deviance increase adolescents' susceptibility to peer pressure.

Problem Behavior Theory. Problem behavior theory explains why youths engage in deviant acts (Jessor and Jessor, 1977). According to this theory, tobacco and alcohol use and unsafe sexual behavior result from an interaction of personal, physiological and genetic, and environmental factors (Jessor, Collins and Jessor, 1972). The theory suggests that some adolescents find deviant acts functional because the acts help them achieve personal goals. For adolescents who are not doing well academically, deviancy may provide a way of achieving social status. Also according to problem behavior theory, youth are more vulnerable to peer pressure when they have few effective coping strategies, few skills to handle social situations, and anxiety about social situations. Although deviant behavior is difficult to prevent if it is functional for youths, that functionalism is vitiated when youths have positive ways of achieving their goals.

Peer Cluster Theory. Peer cluster theory assumes that peer interactions largely determine risk-taking behavior (Oetting and Beauvais, 1986; Oetting and Lynch, in press). Peer clusters include interactions among friends, dating dyads, family constellations and within classrooms, sports teams, and clubs. According to theorists, peer clusters not only account for the presence and type of risk taking among adolescents, but also peer clusters may help youths reduce pressures and influences toward deviance. The therapeutic use of peer clusters in an intervention context may therefore enhance the effects of efforts to reduce adolescents' risks of drug abuse.

Family Networks Theory. The absence of family supports contributes to adolescents' use of tobacco, alcohol, and other drugs (Moncher, Holden and Schinke, 1991; Pandina and Schuele, 1983; Wiess, 1988). Studies have shown an association between harsh parental discipline and chil-

dren's subsequent behavioral problems. Other studies have found a relationship between parental support for health behavior and children's
healthy habits (American Psychological Association, 1993; McLoyd and
Wilson, 1990; Resnick, Chabliss and Blum, 1993). Increased family con-
flict, decreased family management, decreased family rituals, decreased
family cohesion, and low-income have all been related to drug abuse
(Bruce and Emshoff, 1992). Other data have demonstrated the positive
influence of family psychoeducation and expanded social networks on
children's health behavior (McFarlane, 1993). These data suggest the salu-
brious effects of including adolescent's families in a community-based
preventive intervention.

The previous theoretical constructs can inform a skills intervention
approach appropriate for community settings and responsive to high-risk
youth, as described in the following paragraphs.

Skills Interventions

Derived from social learning theory (Bandura, 1977), skills interventions help adolescents prevent problems and promote health through problem solving, coping, and enhanced communication skills (Botvin and
Wills, 1985; Schinke and Gilchrist, 1985). Through the use of established
principles that include modeling, role-playing, coaching, feedback, reinforcement and transfer training, skills-based approaches seek to promote
the acquisition and enhancement of general, personal, and social competence skills to resist negative peer and familial influences and pressures to
use drugs.

Adolescents aged 10 and 11 years offer an ideal developmental period
for targeting drug abuse prevention programs. Beginning at about age 10
and lasting through the middle teen years, youths separate from their
parents, develop independence, establish self-identity, and acquire skills to
function as adults. As youths move from childhood to adolescence, they
experience a decline in parental influence accompanied by an increase in
the influence of peers (Utech and Hoving, 1969). Increased reliance on
peers weakens parental influence and facilitates deviance (Jessor, 1984;
Urberg and Robbins, 1983). Early adolescence is thus a time to experiment
with new patterns of behavior (Bailey, 1992).

In our work, the implementation of a community-based prevention
program involves three strategies. These strategies of implementation can
be adopted by other programs seeking to reduce drug abuse or other
problem behaviors among high-risk youth. The three strategies are: enhance sociocultural relevance of intervention, ensure community owner-
ship, and measure the integrity of the implementation.

Delivered by community-level providers and by peer leaders, community-based skills intervention should address personal, behavioral, and environmental factors to effect prevention competence in high-risk youth via multiple components. Described below, these components might include material on development of self-protective skills and self-efficacy, acquisition of problem solving, coping, and anger management skills, enhancement of social proficiency and resiliency, and social supports for maintaining change.

Problem Solving. Problem-solving skills elements teach youths a 5-step sequence for reducing the likelihood of drug use. Steps in the sequence are: Stop, Options, Decide, Act, and Self-praise. In the Stop step, youths pause and define drug-related problems and their role in solving them. In the second step, Options, youths consider alternatives to behavioral risks associated with drug use. In the Decide step, youths systematically choose the best solution from their options. Act, the fourth step, involves planning and rehearsal.

After planning thoughts, words, and gestures appropriate to the problems, youths practice how to handle personal choices. In the Self-praise step, youths reward themselves for using problem solving.

Coping. Coping content teaches youths cognitive and behavioral strategies to adaptively handle stresses that may trigger drug use. Cognitive skills emphasize internal statements of self-praise and affirmation to help adolescents manage their behavior and reduce their drug risks. Behavioral coping skills teach youths to reward themselves overtly for successful prevention efforts.

Communication and Assertiveness. Communication and assertion skills teach youths how to successfully interact with peers and others to avoid interpersonal triggers for drug use. Youths learn skills to accomplish such different purposes as communicating to achieve an objective, to maintain a relationship, and to gain self-respect. In role-play situations, youths can practice communication skills.

Self-Esteem. This content includes exercises to enhance youths' feelings of self-worth. Exercises focus on ways to build youth's knowledge and awareness of their own special role in the world. For example, youths can complete worksheets that allow them to view themselves relative to milestones in their lives. Exercises in the self-esteem unit also enable youth to learn and apply material on drug abuse risk reduction, health promotion, future goals, and positive habits. Other exercises can provide youth with games to identify their own healthy habits, to describe current and future special skills, and to set life goals in several areas.

Decision Making. Incorporated into decision making are concepts of self-control and values clarification. Decision-making content teaches youths to avoid influences on their behavior, depending on the nature of the influence. For example, youths learn how to recognize when they are faced with unhealthy and risky situations. With equal emphasis, the materials show youths how to take advantage of situations with positive potential.

Exercises in this component enable youths to identify helpful adults in their environments to whom they can turn for assistance. By completing worksheets structured for engaging such assistance, youths learn who can help them and what help those persons can lend when they confront situations that are beyond their abilities. As such, decision-making content contains information on the processes and substance of decision making relative to positive and negative circumstances.

Life Skills Training Community Center Model. An example of skills interventions for community settings is the Life Skills Training (LST) program. Originally designed for school settings, the LST was adapted for after-school community programs. Adaptation of the LST for the community center took into account the varied age group of community center youths, youths' dislike of activities that are too "school-like," and the fact that youths choose to participate in different activities depending on the day. To address these differences, the LST for community centers provides children with a variety of group roles that are appropriate for different ages, rotates skill sessions, integrates several skills into one session, and organizes skills training around nonacademic themes.

In order to avoid drug use, adolescents need to have options for achieving personal goals, such as positive ways of gaining admission to peer groups, of demonstrating independence, and of coping with boredom or anxiety. The LST uses community service projects to teach individual skills and also to provide opportunities for meaningful roles in the community. These opportunities can include: working in day care centers, running errands for the elderly, turning graffiti covered walls into murals, organizing a tutoring service for younger children, collecting food for the homeless, and turning abandoned vacant lots into community gardens.

Groups meet at least once a week for approximately 2 hours each time. The meetings are used for (1) skills training, (2) discussion of project goals and progress, and (3) activities geared towards meeting those goals. Intervention providers weave the discussion and practice of the particular skills lesson into the work on the community projects.

Community service activities help to attract and retain participants, promote a sense of group identity and group efficacy, and underscore the fact that there are positive alternatives to drug use. What is more, these activities are a natural vehicle for skills training. Core components of the competence enhancement approach to drug prevention (including problem solving, coping, and decision making, as described previously, as well as self-image, goal-setting, social skills, general assertive skills and drug resistance skills) are presented in each activity.

In a newsletter activity, for example, participants decided to create a biography of a community figure for each issue of the newsletter. As part of this biography, they developed and practiced an interview each week. They assumed various roles as they "worked the bugs out" of the interview. During this process there was an ideal opportunity to demonstrate and practice communication skills (e.g., eye contact, avoiding misunderstandings), social skills (e.g., how to keep a conversation going), and assertiveness skills (e.g., how to express an opinion). These role plays allow discussion, demonstration, and practice of the important personal and social skills that are taught in the LST program. Thus, at every opportunity during group interactions, competence enhancement concepts are applied and reinforced by the intervention providers.

Intervention providers are recreational workers from community agencies who are trained in competence enhancement skills. These providers implement the program with youth groups during regular after-school sessions. Adolescents and their parent(s) sign up for the LST program in the same manner as they do for other recreational programs provided by the center. Skills are presented in rotation in order to reach those youths who do not attend groups consistently. Participants who attend regularly act as peer leaders and assist the group leader in demonstrating skills and organizing activities.

Parent Involvement

Parent involvement can strengthen youths' learning through positive family interactions that support risk reduction efforts (Hawkins, Catalano and Miller, 1992; Hawkins et al., 1992). Parents can include natural parents and other significant adult members of youths' lives. Interactive exercises should encourage parent-child communication not only around risk reduction content, but also around shared enjoyable activities. Shared parent-child exercises can be introduced during monthly family sessions. Risk-reduction research has found family sessions more effective than exercises completed at home for increasing ethnic-racial minority parent participation and for changing youths' behavior (Perry, 1993).

In our previous work with family interventions, we found that parents valued activities focused on their needs, not only on their children's needs (Moncher, 1991). To that end, parent intervention might include events exclusively for youths' parents. Such parent sessions should have provisions for child care and transportation reimbursements. Parenting workshops might encompass child-management skills (e.g., negotiation, positive reinforcement) and ideas to help youths avoid tobacco, alcohol, and other drug use. For example, because low levels of parental support and weak parental sanctions against using tobacco and alcohol are related to adolescent drug use (Jessor and Jessor, 1977), parents can practice communicating strong, consistent messages about abstinence from tobacco and alcohol use to their children. Parents might also learn that effective parenting consists of being warm toward one's children, engaging in a high degree of give-and-take, offering rational explanations of rules and limits, and affirming their children's qualities coupled with setting clear standards for conduct (Baumrind, 1978).

Although generalizations are hazardous in describing such a varied population as parents of high-risk youth, our prior data suggests that these parents might be inordinately occupied with providing for their households and thus might have limited time for working with their children around drug prevention goals. Admittedly, many drug abuse prevention activities presume a commitment of parents that may not always be possible. But through the help of focus groups and consultants, the parent involvement component can be crafted to accommodate many parenting styles. For example, if key figures in the community believe that parent attendance at intervention sessions is unrealistic, workbook or video instruction can be created for shared parent-youth activities at home.

Community Involvement

Aside from the obvious ethical and theoretical advantages of involving the community in an intervention, there are a number of practical benefits of involving the community in the implementation of any intervention. With community participation, the study requires less staff, is more likely to have relevance to the community, and is more likely to be a lasting force within the community.

Our experience has taught us that community-based health promotion efforts which fail to directly address the community as part of the larger sociopolitical context are unlikely to be successful. Such narrowly focused efforts are liable to fail at three key points: initial outreach and entry into the community, program implementation, and institutionalization. Designing a curriculum for community-based prevention studies should be a collaborative effort with target members of the community. Parents, youth, community leaders, school staff, and human service workers can all take part in curriculum development. We have found that without the approval of such community representatives, health promotion and risk reduction efforts designed for youths in community settings are less likely to succeed.

As a first step in a community-based prevention intervention study, the research team should contact target community figures and urban organizations to invite their participation in the project. A meeting with key community figures to discuss effective ways to implement the prevention project in the target community is recommended. At this meeting, researchers can present current prevention research and health promotion strategies for the target population. Then community representatives can voice their health concerns and opinions about the strengths and weaknesses of current prevention programs.

Community representatives can contribute to the intervention in several ways. In our past work with drug abuse prevention and Native American youth, for example, community representatives helped highlight how the commercialization of tobacco had overshadowed its traditional ceremonial use (Schinke, Singer, Cole and Contento, in press). Collaborating community representatives can help emphasize cultural awareness within the intervention and can ensure accurate and sensitive cultural information.

Concurrent with skills and parent components, community involvement strategies extend drug prevention activities into high-risk youths' neighborhoods and everyday environments. That extension occurs as subjects plan and execute events that involve extended family members, neighborhood residents, and community members. These events might include community meetings, poster-making exercises, and problem-solving contests.

Community meetings take place at collaborating sites. Besides youths and intervention providers, these meetings should include youths' extended kinship network members, community residents, and neighbors. Intervention delivery agents encourage youths to invite community leaders (e.g., local politicians, elected and government officials, and clergy), professionals, merchants and business representatives, and extended family members (including unrelated neighbors) to the meetings.

Intervention leaders and youths plan meetings, which should involve arranging for the provision of child care for community participants. After on-site staff explain the theme for each community meeting, youths develop and rehearse an agenda. For example, youths might present skits, lead group discussions, and show audio-visual materials on drug prevention.

Presentations demonstrate what youths know about drug abuse risk reduction and how those in attendance can help youths avoid behavioral risks associated with drugs. Each participant receives a written summary of steps covered at the meeting to help youths avoid risky behaviors associated with drug use.

Interpersonal communication posters engage youths in designing, creating, and distributing throughout their neighborhoods and communities posters about preventing drug use. Posters remind community members that everyone is responsible for assisting youths in avoiding life-style behaviors associated with drugs. In their poster designs, youths incorporate landmarks, language, and symbols that have meaning for them. Youths exhibit the posters throughout their neighborhoods in stores, community centers, and other public places. Intervention agents and peer leaders visit each poster display, take photographs of the posters, and display the photographs at each community site.

A problem-solving contest begins with a series of assignments related to a hypothetical youth who has encountered a problem related to drug risks. Next, team members apply problem-solving steps to plan how those hypothetical persons will resolve their problems and reduce their risks. The application of each step brings youths into contact with community members. Youths analyze and apply outside information they gather within a problem-solving format.

Concurrently, the contest exposes community members to intervention as youths collect information, conduct interviews, and draw on resources beyond the community site. Youths earn points for each piece of information they gather and for each community member with whom they interact relative to drug risks. For example, team members gain points for the options they generate via resources to resolve the hypothetical situation posed by another team. Teams receive additional points for enlisting the help of neighbors, community members, health and human services professionals, and civic leaders in their problem-solving efforts.

COMMUNITY-BASED STUDY FINDINGS

The authors have conducted community-based studies with intervention for high-risk youth similar to the one described above (Moncher and Schinke, 1994; Schinke and Cole, 1995; Schinke, Jansen, Kennedy and Shi, 1994; Schinke, Moncher and Singer, in press; Schinke et al., 1992; Schinke et al., 1992; Schinke et al., in press). These studies have taught us several lessons. A prevention study, for example, with Native American youth to prevent cancers associated with drug use and diet taught us important lessons about site and subject recruitment methods with Native American youth. Recruitment interviews with participating community sites led us to believe that collaborating Native American agencies served sufficient numbers of Native American youths in our target age range. We later discovered that many of these sites' services were sporadic and typically geared to adults rather than children. Because no regular recreational or social activities for children were offered, families with children were sometimes unacquainted with the organization and thus leery of participating in the intervention.

In addition, although the Native American organizations reported accurately the number of Native American youth they serve annually, the numbers shrink and swell depending on the time of year. Many of the Native Americans served by our urban sites spend considerable time each year on their native reservations and were thus unavailable at various times throughout intervention delivery. Although these issues may seem unique to Native American culture, we have encountered similar recruitment problems in our work with other community-based studies.

In a community-based study with economically disadvantaged youth in the Northeast, for example, we found that the heterogeneity of the study sample confounded our study procedures (Schinke et al., 1994). Unlike a classroom, the community agencies from which we drew our study sample served youths aged from 6 to 16 years. Such a broad age range had implications for our developing one responsive intervention curricula. Children aged 6 years are obviously quite different cognitively and emotionally than youths who are 16 years. Yet, creating multiple curricula was beyond the scope of our study.

Also in this study and in numerous other community-based studies that we have conducted, we found that youths are loath to complete written measurement instruments. Outside of school, youths seem particularly opposed to completing paper and pencil measurement instruments. To avoid this problem, we have used measures that rely on videotape, or that involve interactive computer technologies, whenever possible. In addition, we make every effort to keep written measures as simple and as brief as possible.

Defining the sections of the community to target is also important. In a drug abuse prevention study based in Seguin and San Antonio, Texas, for example, we initially planned to target the entire community, including all of its schools and major mass media. Nor did we subdivide the community into various cultural subgroups. But in this racially and ethnically segregated community, the geographically defined community had little in common with the cultural community. Despite the intervention's intent to address the whole community, the project gradually became identified as an exclusively Hispanic project. As a result, preexisting social networks in the community were often negative rather than positive forces.

Yet, the positive effects of community-based prevention are many. In a study of Boys & Girls Clubs that had drug abuse prevention programs and were based in public housing developments, we found that, for adults and youths alike, Boys & Girls Clubs appear to be associated with an overall reduction in drug abuse, drug trafficking, and other drug-related criminal activity (Schinke et al., 1992). Illustrative data from that study, for example, show that crack cocaine use decreased in public housing developments with Boys & Girls Clubs, but increased in the control public housing developments. From data collected in two of the cities with index public housing developments, we found that 13% fewer police reports on juvenile criminal activity were filed in beats that covered the housing developments with Boys & Girls Clubs compared to beats that covered the housing developments that did not have Boys & Girls Clubs.

Boys & Girls Club programs appear to improve the physical quality of life in housing developments, which seems to have boosted the morale of the development's residents and authority figures in the community. Through interviews, members of the evaluation team discovered that the presence of BGCs in housing developments encourages residents to organize and improve their community. BGCs stimulate communication between housing development residents, the police, housing authority managing personnel, and other community groups. The increase in communication seems to have enriched the social quality of life in the housing developments. This informal interaction and communication is perhaps the most important effect of the BGCs and it is also the most difficult to measure.

CONCLUSION

Increasingly, prevention researchers are discovering that youth who are living below the Federal poverty line are at high risk for encountering future and life-long problems with drugs, including alcohol and tobacco. In response to that discovery, drug abuse preventive interventions must be developed expressly for such high-risk youth. Those interventions will wisely address community as well as parental and developmental factors that influence drug use among high-risk youth.

Community-based skills interventions to prevent drug use include elements on drug use facts, problem-solving, coping, communication, and decision-making skills. As important, these interventions incorporate the community and family in both intervention development and intervention implementation. Admittedly, this prevention approach and its application has limitations. Involving subjects' communities and their parents takes extraordinary time and effort. Many parents simply do not have the time to participate in the activities that preventive skills intervention requires. Yet, their involvement is critical to the successful outcome of the prevention project. Similarly, youths find recruiting community members formidable and occasionally disappointing; some community members promise to participate, and then do not attend. Developing an intervention that is culturally relevant for every ethnic-racial minority group represented in the study population is also challenging.

Still, on the balance, the skills intervention approach advocated here has much to recommend it for youth at high risk for problems associated with drug and other drug abuse. Additional research will refine and expand this prevention approach so that it ultimately reaches all of the high-risk youth who can benefit from aggressive efforts to prevent drug use and abuse in the community.

REFERENCES

American Psychological Association. (1993). *Violence and youth: Psychology's response* (Vol. 1. Summary Report of the American Psychological Association Commission on Violence and Youth). Washington, DC: American Psychological Association.

Bailey, S. L. (1992). Adolescents' multisubstance use patterns: The role of heavy alcohol and cigarette use. *American Journal of Public Health, 82*, 1220-1224.

Bambade, S., & Chalmers, D. (1991). Co-victimization of African-American children who witness violence: Effects on cognitive, emotional, and behavioral development. *Journal of National Medical Association, 83*(3), 233-238.

Bandura, A. (1977). *Social learning theory.* Englewood Cliffs, NJ: Prentice-Hall.

Baumrind, D. (1978). Parental disciplinary patterns and social competence in youth. *Youth and Society, 9*, 239-276.

Botvin, G. J., & Wills, T. A. (1985). Personal and social skills training: Cognitive-behavioral approaches to substance abuse prevention. In C. Bell & R. Battjes (Eds.), *Prevention research: Deterring drug abuse among children and adolescents, NIDA Research Monograph Series.* Washington, DC: U. S. Government Printing Office.

Bruce, C., & Emshoff, J. (1992). The Super II Program: An early intervention program. *Journal of Community Psychology* (OSAP Special Issue), 10-21.

Center for the Study of Social Policy. (1986). The "flip-side" of black families headed by women: The economic status of black men. In R. Staples (Ed.), *The black family: Essays and studies* (pp. 232-238). Belmont, CA: Wadsworth.

Cloward, R., & Ohlin, L. (1960). *Delinquency and opportunity.* New York: Free Press.

Department of Health and Human Services. (1985). *Report of the Secretary's Task Force on Black and Minority Health.* Washington, DC: Author.

Dusenbury, L., Kerner, J. F., Baker, E., Botvin, G., James-Ortiz, S., & Zauber, A. (1992). Predictors of smoking prevalence among New York Latino youth. *American Journal of Public Health, 82*, 55-58.

Elliot, D., Ageton, S., & Canter, R. (1979). An integrated theoretical perspective on delinquent behavior. *Journal of Research in Crime and Delinquency, 16*, 3-27.

Flay, B. R. (1985). Psychosocial approaches to smoking prevention: A review of the findings. *Health Psychology, 4*, 449-488.

Fraser, M., & Kohlert, N. (1988). Substance abuse and public policy. *Social Service Review, 62*(1), 103-125.

Goplerud, E. (1991). *Breaking new ground for youth at risk: Program summaries* (ADAMHA. OSAP Technical Report-1.): U. S. Dept. of Health and Human Services: Public Health Service.

Greenwald, P., Cullen, J. W., & McKenna, J. W. (1987). Cancer prevention and control: From research through applications. *Journal of the National Cancer Institute, 79*, 389-400.

Hawkins, J. D., Catalano, R. F., & Miller, J. Y. (1992). Risk and protective factors for alcohol and other drug problems in adolescence and early childhood: Implications for substance abuse prevention. *Psychological Bulletin, 112*(1), 103-115.

Hawkins, J. D., Catalano, R. F., Morrison, D. M., O'Donnell, J., Abbott, R. D., & Day, L. E. (1992). The Seattle social development project: Effects of the first four years on protective factors and problem behaviors. In J. McCord & R. Tremblay (Eds.), *The prevention of antisocial behavior in children* (pp. 139-161). New York: Guilford.

Hechinger, F. M. (1992). *Fateful choices: Healthy youth for the 21st century.* New York: Carnegie Corporation.

Hiatt, R. A., Klatsky, A. L., & Armstrong, M. A. (1988). Alcohol consumption and the risk of breast cancer in a prepaid health plan. *Cancer Research, 48*, 2284-2287.

Hirschi, T. (1969). *Causes of delinquency.* Berkeley: University of California Press.

Institute of Medicine. (1991). *Broadening the base of treatment for alcohol problems.* Washington, DC: National Academy Press.

Jessor, R. (1984). Adolescent development and behavioral health. In J. D. Matarazzo, S. M. Weiss, J. A. Herd, N. E. Miller, & S. M. Weiss (Eds.), *Behavioral health* (pp. 69-90). New York: John Wiley.

Jessor, R., Collins, M. I., & Jessor, S. L. (1972). On becoming a drinker. *Annual of the New York Academy of Sciences, 197*, 199-213.

Jessor, R., & Jessor, S. L. (1977). *Problem behavior & psychosocial development.* New York: Academic Press.

Johnson, J. (1990). Preventive interventions for children at risk: Introduction. *International Journal of the Addictions, 25*, 429-434.

Johnston, L. D., O'Malley, P. M., & Bachman, J. G. (1995). *National Survey*

Results on Drug Use from the Monitoring the Future Study, 1975-1994. Vol. I Secondary School Students. Rockville, MD: National Institute on Drug Abuse.

McFarlane, W. R. (1993). *The multiple family group, psychoeducation and maintenance medication in the treatment of schizophrenia: Psychiatric outcomes in a multi-site trial.*

McKay, J. R., Murphy, R. T., McGuire, J., Rivinus, T. R., & Maisto, S. A. (1992). Incarcerated adolescents' attributions for drug and alcohol use. *Addictive Behaviors, 17,* 227-235.

McLoyd, V., & Wilson, L. (1990). Maternal behavior, social support, and economic conditions as predictors of distress in children. In W. Damon (Ed.), *New directions for child development* (pp. 49-71). San Francisco: Jossey-Bass.

Moncher, M. S. (1991). *Process and outcome evaluation of intervention curriculum to increase parent involvement with students in character development program.* Unpublished Doctoral dissertation (1990), Columbia University.

Moncher, M. S., Holden, G. W., & Schinke, S. P. (1991). Psychosocial correlates of substance abuse among youth: A review of current etiological constructs. *International Journal of the Addictions, 26,* 377-414.

Moncher, M. S., & Schinke, S. P. (1994). Group intervention to prevent tobacco use among Native American youth. *Research on Social Work Practice, 4,* 160-171.

National Institute on Drug Abuse. (1985). *Drug use among American high school students, college students, and other young adults.* Rockville, MD: Government Printing Office.

National Substance Abuse Institute. (1991). *Strategies to control tobacco use in the United States.* Bethesda, MD: National Substance Abuse Institute.

Oetting, E., & Beauvais, F. (1986). Peer cluster theory: Drugs and the adolescent. *Journal of Counseling Development, 65*(1), 17-22.

Oetting, E. R., & Lynch, R. S. (in press). Peers and the prevention of adolescent drug use. In Z. Amsel & B. Bukoski (Eds.), *Handbook for drug abuse prevention, theory and practice.* New York: Plenum.

Pandina, R. T., & Schuele, J. A. (1983). Psychosocial correlates of alcohol and drug use of adolescent students and adolescents in treatment. *Journal of Studies on Alcohol, 44,* 950-973.

Pavkov, T. W., McGovern, M. P., & Geffner, E. S. (1993). Problem severity and symptomatology among substance misusers: Differences between African-Americans and Caucasians. *International Journal of the Addictions, 28,* 909-922.

Pentz, M. A. (1983). Prevention of adolescent substance abuse through social skills. In T. J. Glynn, C. G. Leukefeld, & J. P. Ludford (Eds.), *Preventing adolescent drug abuse: Intervention strategies.* Washington, DC: U. S. Government Printing Office.

Perry, C. (1993). *Review of CATCH findings on CVD risk reduction in urban and rural settings.* New York: Cornell University Medical College.

Resnick, M. D., Chabliss, S. A., & Blum, R. W. (1993). Health and risk behaviors of urban adolescent males involved in pregnancy. *Families in Society, 74,* 366-374.

Schinke, S. P., Bebel, M. Y., Orlandi, M. A., & Botvin, G. J. (1988). Prevention strategies for vulnerable pupils. *Urban Education, 22,* 510-519.

Schinke, S. P., & Cole, K. C. (1995). Methodological issues in conducting alcohol abuse prevention research in ethnic communities. In P. A. Langton (Ed.), *Preventing alcohol-related problems in ethnic communities* (pp. 129-147). Rockville, MD: Substance Abuse and Mental Services Administration.

Schinke, S. P., & Gilchrist, L. D. (1984). *Life skills counseling with adolescents.* Baltimore, MD: University Park.

Schinke, S. P., & Gilchrist, L. D. (1985). Preventing substance abuse with children and adolescents. *Journal of Consulting and Clinical Psychology, 53,* 598-602.

Schinke, S. P., Jansen, M., Kennedy, E., & Shi, Q. (1994). Reducing risk taking behavior among vulnerable youth: An intervention outcome study. *Family and Community Health, 16*(4), 49-56.

Schinke, S. P., Moncher, M. S., & Singer, B. R. (in press). Native American youths and cancer risk reduction: Effects of software intervention. *Journal of Adolescent Health.*

Schinke, S. P., Orlandi, M. A., & Cole, K. C. (1992). Boys and girls clubs in public housing developments: Prevention services for youth at risk. *Journal of Community Psychology, 28,* 118-128.

Schinke, S. P., Orlandi, M. A., Vaccaro, D., Espinoza, R., McAlister, A., & Botvin, G. J. (1992). Substance use among Hispanic and non-Hispanic adolescents. *Addictive Behaviors, 17,* 117-124.

Schinke, S. P., Singer, B., Cole, K., & Contento, I. R. (in press). Reducing cancer risks among Native American adolescents: Cultural issues, intervention strategies, and baseline findings. *Preventive Medicine.*

Urberg, & Robbins, R. (1983). *Adolescent invulnerability.* Unpublished manuscript. Detroit, MI: Wayne State University.

U. S. Congress Office of Technology Assessment. (1986). *Children's mental health: Problems and services—A background paper (OTA-BP-H-33).* Washington, DC: U. S. Government Printing Office.

U. S. Congress Office of Technology Assessment. (1991). *Adolescent health. (OTA-H-468).* Washington, DC: U. S. Government Printing Office.

U. S. Department of Health and Human Services. (1990). *Healthy people 2000: National health promotion and disease prevention objectives.* Washington, DC: U. S. Department of Health and Human Services.

Utech, D., & Hoving, K. L. (1969). Parents and peers as competing influences in the decisions on children of differing ages. *Journal of Social Psychology, 78,* 267-274.

Walter, H., Vaughan, R. D., Gladis, M. M., Ragin, D. F., Kasen, S., & Cohall, A. T. (1992). Factors associated with AIDS risk behaviors among high school students in an AIDS epicenter. *American Journal of Public Health, 82,* 528-532.

Walter, H. J., Vaughan, R. D., & Cohall, A. T. (1991). Risk factors for substance use among high school students: Implications for prevention. *Journal of the American Academy of Child and Adolescent Psychiatry, 30,* 556-562.

Wiess, H. B. (1988). Family support and education programs: Working through ecological theories of human development. In H. B. Wiess & F. H. Jacobs (Eds.), *Evaluating family programs* (pp. 3-36). New York: Aldine De Gruyter.

Zigler, E., Taussig, C., & Black, K. (1992). Early childhood intervention. *American Psychologist, 47,* 997-1006.

Risk Factors for Alcohol Use Among Inner-City Minority Youth: A Comparative Analysis of Youth Living in Public and Conventional Housing

Christopher Williams
Lawrence M. Scheier
Gilbert J. Botvin
Eli Baker
Nicole Miller

SUMMARY. National survey data indicate that drug use among our nation's secondary school youth is once again on the rise. Nowhere is this concern more dramatic than with inner-city youth who seem disproportionately affected by the risks associated with drug use. Ur-

Christopher Williams, PhD, Lawrence M. Scheier, PhD, Gilbert J. Botvin, PhD, Eli Baker, PhD, and Nicole Miller, MPH, are affiliated with the Institute for Prevention Research, Cornell University Medical College, 411 East 69th Street, New York, NY 10021.

Address correspondence to Christopher Williams, PhD, Institute for Prevention Research, Department of Public Health, Cornell University Medical College, 411 East 69th Street, KB 201, New York, NY 10021.

Preparation of this article was partially supported by a research grant to Gilbert J. Botvin (P50DA-7656) and a FIRST Award to Lawrence M. Scheier (R29-DA08909-03) from the National Institute on Drug Abuse.

[Haworth co-indexing entry note]: "Risk Factors for Alcohol Use Among Inner-City Minority Youth: A Comparative Analysis of Youth Living in Public and Conventional Housing." Williams, Christopher et al. Co-published simultaneously in *Journal of Child & Adolescent Substance Abuse* (The Haworth Press, Inc.) Vol. 6, No. 1, 1997, pp. 69-89; and: *The Etiology and Prevention of Drug Abuse Among Minority Youth* (ed: Gilbert J. Botvin, and Steven Schinke) The Haworth Press, Inc., 1997, pp. 69-89. Single or multiple copies of this article are available for a fee from The Haworth Document Delivery Service [1-800-342-9678, 9:00 a.m. - 5:00 p.m. (EST). E-mail address: getinfo@ haworth.com].

ban youth residing in public housing developments may be extremely vulnerable as a result of their exposure to high rates of crime, unrelenting poverty, and drug use. To better understand the role of public housing conditions in the etiology of adolescent drug use, we examined a sample of youth living in housing developments and youth living in conventional housing. Correlates and predictors of alcohol and drug use included measures of cognitive efficacy, social influences, normative expectations, drug-refusal skills, family management, psychological distress, and alcohol-related expectancies. Overall, there were few significant mean differences in psychosocial functioning or drug behavior for the two groups. Hierarchical moderated multiple regression analyses indicated that public housing status buffered against the negative effects of high levels of perceived alcohol availability on drinking behavior, whereas youth living in conventional housing with high grades reported lower alcohol involvement. Findings are discussed in terms of their implications for developing effective prevention approaches targeting urban youth residing in public housing. *[Article copies available for a fee from The Haworth Document Delivery Service: 1-800-342-9678. E-mail address: getinfo@haworth.com]*

KEYWORDS. Alcohol Use, Minority Youth, Public Housing Developments, Inner-Cities

Urban life across America is often characterized by conditions of economic blight and social disorganization. Prevalence rates for crime are highest among inner-cities (Statistical Abstracts of the United States, 1995) and trend data for arrest records among inner-cities show increases in all major crime categories. Coupled with these indicators, labor statistics reveal that unemployment is highest among urban locales (Statistical Abstracts of the United States, 1995). In New York City, for example, only 55.5% of its residents reported working in 1994, compared with 66.6% in the United States and 64.1% in the Northeast region (Social Indicators, 1995). Nowhere are the adverse economic and social conditions more apparent than in inner-city housing developments. Because they are often geographically separated from economically thriving commercial centers, public housing developments form a catchment area for low-income residents creating a magnet for unemployment and crime. Beset with poverty and its associated difficulties, many inner-city residents turn to drugs as a form of coping.

The adverse effects of persistent poverty, high unemployment, and low rates of social mobility may also extend to inner-city youth. Nationwide survey data obtained from secondary school students, for example, indicate that there are higher rates of adolescent drug use among inner-cities compared to rural or suburban locations (Johnston, O'Malley, and Bachman, 1994). The aftershocks of social strain may also extend to other domains of functioning among inner-city youth as evidenced by higher dropout rates (Figueira-McDonough, 1992), higher rates of teenage pregnancy (Danziger, 1995), increased prevalence of criminal and delinquent behavior (Elliot, Huizinga, and Menard, 1989) and poor socioemotional functioning (e.g., Spencer, Brookins, and Allen, 1985).

More often than not, subsidized housing projects provide a breeding ground for many of the problems besetting inner-city youth. Public housing developments offer crowded residences with high concentrations of disadvantaged minorities and are located in racially segregated neighborhoods characterized by urban blight. Moreover, youthful occupants of housing developments lack protection from the adverse socioeconomic conditions that encourage delinquency among adult residents. Durant, Pendergrast, and Cadenhead (1994), for example, reported that exposure to violence, being victimized in the home and community, and experiencing feelings of hopelessness predicted domestic problems and gang-related fighting among youth living in housing developments. Along these lines, Dembo and his colleagues (Dembo, Allen, Farrow, Schmeidler, and Burgos, 1985; Dembo, Burgos, Des Jarlais, and Schmeidler, 1979; Dembo, Schmeidler, Burgos, and Taylor, 1985) have shown that perceived drug availability is associated with self-reported drug use among inner-city minority youth. Based on several studies that concentrated on the role of environmental factors in promoting drug use, these authors conclude that drug use among youth residing in tough, gang-oriented neighborhoods represents a dynamic of affirmation that helps lift these youth from feelings of despair to a more positive social context. Farrell, Danish, and Howard (1992) reported that environmental variables (e.g., perceived employment opportunities and trouble with police) were some of the strongest predictors of self-reported drug use among a sample of predominantly inner-city and economically disadvantaged African-American youth. Although there is not a specific body of literature on the effects of adolescents living in inner-city public housing developments, there exists a substantial body of empirical knowledge that suggests that high concentrations of poverty, blocked access to gainful employment (McLoyd, 1995), exposure to violence and drug-related activities (Hawkins, Catalano, and Miller, 1992) all lead to poor behavioral and emotional outcomes for children and adolescents. Findings from these studies and others suggest that public housing youth, in particular, may be at increased risk because specific contextual features of the surrounding community such as unemployment and low rates of economic and social mobility may foster increased rates of crime and delinquency.

Furthermore, recent statistics from New York City reveal that residents of public housing developments are exposed to more violent and drug-related crime than residents from adjacent neighborhoods (New York City Housing Authority, 1994). Facing deleterious conditions that spawn antisocial behavior, many of these youth turn to drugs as a means of escape from harsh living conditions. Despite recent attempts to understand relations between risk and drug use among inner-city youth (e.g., Brook, Lukoff, and Whiteman, 1977; Brunswick and Messeri, 1983-84; Epstein, Botvin, Diaz, and Schinke, 1994), few of these studies have examined precisely how environmental conditions such as living situations (i.e., public subsidized housing) among inner-city minority youth may influence drug use.

HOUSING DEVELOPMENTS AS PROTECTIVE ENVIRONMENTS

Despite claims that youth living in public housing are at high risk for negative behavioral and emotional outcomes (Spencer, Brookins, and Allen, 1985), an emerging body of qualitative research suggests that several protective mechanisms may reduce delinquency among public housing youth. Pressed by dire economic circumstances and high rates of crime, parents of these youth may form protective enclaves with heightened community activity. Examples of this activity include parent-initiated security patrols, efforts to create safe playgrounds, and community activism to reduce crime (McLaughlin, Irby, and Langman, 1994; Vergara, 1989). Several studies have shown increased parental monitoring (Williams and Kornblum, 1995), stringent curfews, and high security in recreational areas for children are all features of housing developments that can successfully reduce crime and drug use (McLaughlin et al., 1994). It is also important to consider, based on studies of risk and resilience (Garmezy, 1985), that individuals vary in their ability to resist the vicissitudes of inner-city life. Even the most abject conditions of poverty and social chaos do not necessarily propel every youth into a life of drug abuse and crime.

IMPORTANCE OF THE CURRENT STUDY

As there is a lack of information that details how specific living conditions may affect risk for drug use and related problem behaviors, further studies are required that examine the contribution of environmental features to early-stage drug use. Both society and the high-risk individuals residing in these environments can benefit from targeted interventions that reduce precocious drug use. Additionally, effective and rational development of these interventions requires empirical knowledge of risk processes. To learn more about drug use etiology and inner-city housing status, we conducted a study of youth residing in inner-city subsidized (public) housing developments and a sample of demographically matched youth residing in nonsubsidized (conventional) housing. We specifically focused on alcohol consumption because alcohol was the most prevalently used drug and because the alcohol use data provided sufficient variation for robust parameter estimation using regression techniques. Several dimensions of psychosocial risk were assessed including social influences (i.e., peer models and normative expectations), alcohol expectancies (perceived consequences) and knowledge (facts about alcohol), social skills (e.g., communication and assertiveness skills), personal competence (e.g., decision-making and self-management skills), psychosocial functioning (i.e., depression and self-esteem), and measures of social control (e.g., absenteeism, church attendance, grades). The dimensions of risk included in this study were organized into conceptual domains similar to those suggested by other researchers (e.g., Petraitis, Flay, and Miller, 1995). While housing developments have often been utilized as sites for examining drug behaviors among adults, a unique and important aspect of the present study is that it examines the impact of housing status on drug use among minority youth.

METHOD

Sample

Data for the current study were obtained as part of an ongoing prospective investigation of drug abuse etiology and prevention with inner-city minority youth. Only individuals not assigned to receive a preventive intervention were eligible for inclusion in this study. A subsample of 700 minority youth who reported that they lived in public subsidized housing developments in the New York metropolitan area was selected for inclusion in the study. A second subsample of 700 minority youths who reported that they lived in conventional housing was randomly selected from the remaining sample as a matched comparison group. Both samples were then further selected to include African-American and Hispanic students. A third and quite small ethnic group included students of mixed origin and subsequent analyses revealed no significant differences between the minority and "other" categories and youth in this category were eliminated.

The public housing sample consisted of both middle income (n = 268) and low income housing residents based on federal guidelines (n = 356). Descriptive analyses between these two groups revealed few significant differences in any of the major demographic, psychological, and behavioral measures. Therefore for subsequent analyses, the low and middle income public housing groups were collapsed into one group. The resultant public housing sample included 622 youths (169 Hispanic and 453 African-American, 42% male). The matched comparison group included 642 conventional housing youth (90 Hispanic, and 552 African-American, 46% male). Proportional analyses indicated no differential composition based on gender for the two samples. Approximately half of the students in both groups lived in single-parent, female-headed households (54.3% and 50.7% public housing versus conventional housing groups, respectively). Underscoring the disadvantaged status of these youths, 64.2% of both groups reported that they received lunch free or at reduced (subsidized) prices. Passive consent procedures were used and less than 1% of the entire baseline pretest sample refused participation.

Behavioral, Attitudinal, and Psychosocial Measures

Items included in the survey assessed intra- and interpersonal functioning as well as a variety of attitudes, intentions, and behaviors related to alcohol (and other drug) use. Frequency of alcohol (beer, wine, and hard liquor) use was assessed by one item ("About how often (if ever) do you drink beer, wine coolers or hard liquor") with responses ranging from "never" (1) to "more than once a day" (9). With an identical response scale, a single item assessed drunkenness ("About how often do you drink until you get drunk"). A single item assessed quantity of alcohol consumption ("If you drink alcohol, how much do you usually drink each time you drink") with responses ranging from "I don't drink" (1) to "more than 6 drinks" (6). These three behavioral items were combined into a single composite score with higher scores indicating greater alcohol involvement.

Using a method proposed by Lu (1974) and subsequently revised by Douglass and Khavari (1982), we used a percentile indexed method to calibrate the measure of alcohol involvement so that less frequent but more severe drinking behaviors (i.e., drunkenness) are given a greater relative weight in the composite measure. In this manner, the indexed value for a student indicating a raw score of 3 on a six-point scale would arithmetically include the frequency of students selecting 1 and 2 and the halved frequency choosing 3 to the same question divided by the total N of youth responding to the item. Indexing was conducted at the item level prior to forming the composite score.

Perceived social influences including perceived best friend ("How many of your friends do you think drink") and peer ("How many people your age do you think drink") alcohol use were rated on a five-point scale ranging from "none" (1) to "all or almost all" (5). Perceived adult alcohol use ("How many adults do you think drink") was also rated on the same five-point scale.

Extensive psychometric information is available for the multi-item scales in both Botvin (1993) and Scheier and Botvin (1995). Also, Scheier and Botvin (this volume) provide estimates of internal consistency for the full baseline sample (from which this select sample was drawn) for identical measures. In general, Cronbach alphas ranged from a low .52 for task persistence (e.g., "If something is really difficult, I get frustrated and quit") to .91 for ethnic identity (e.g., "I have a lot of pride in my ethnic group and its accomplishments").

For the purpose of conducting subsequent analyses, we grouped the psychosocial measures into conceptually and theoretically meaningful clusters of risk factors. This grouping was based, in part, on recent reviews that have delineated the most prominent theories of adolescent drug use (Petraitis, Flay, and Miller, 1995). We used three categories of risk including: cognitive-affective risk (e.g., social outcome expectancies and drug knowledge measures), social/environmental risk (e.g., peer and friends' influence, perceived availability of alcohol, and perceived adult alcohol use), and psychosocial risk, the latter category including a wide array of measures of inter- and intrapersonal functioning (i.e., cognitive self-management, decision-making skills, task persistence, self-reinforcement, self-esteem, family management, school bonding, antisocial behavior, sensation-seeking, ethnic identity, and anxious and depressive symptoms).

Additional measures included age, gender, nuclear family status (intact versus other) and ethnic (racial) self-identification. A single item queried students about their means of obtaining lunch (e.g., subsidized, free lunch or bring lunch from home) and is used as an index for socioeconomic status. Students also provided self-reported grades, church attendance, and school absenteeism.

Data Analysis

The primary hypothesis of this study is that housing status (public or conventional) is a moderator of the relationship of psychosocial risk and drug use, and would vary in its effect on alcohol consumption depending on which condition of vulnerability was being examined. Following analytic conventions proposed by Baron and Kenny (1986), we used moderated multiple regression with hierarchical inclusion to test for buffering effects. Using this approach, a composite measure of alcohol (frequency, intensity, and drunkenness) was regressed on each of the risk predictors, followed by the inclusion of the moderator (housing status) and subsequently an interaction term representing the cross-product of the predictor and moderator. A significant interaction term, controlling for the main effects of risk and housing status, indicates a buffering or conditional effect. Moderator or buffering effects usually take on the form of crossover, disordinal, or fan-shaped regression lines underscoring the change in slope at each level of the continuous predictor. Following recommendations made by Aiken and West (1991), we plotted predicted outcome scores corresponding to the simple main effects for each level of the moderator variable. This method provides a useful graphical means of detecting significant crossover or disordinal interactions.

RESULTS

Prevalence Rates of Alcohol Consumption

Based on a combined sample of youth living in public housing and conventional housing, slightly under one-third of these youth reported some use of alcohol. Using a use/nonuse distinction, public housing and conventional housing youth did not significantly differ in the proportion of alcohol users. There were also no significant differences between public and conventional housing youth in mean level of alcohol consumption, intensity of use, or self-reported drunkenness. We also examined self-reported use of cigarettes and marijuana among non-abstaining youth. Among self-reported alcohol users, housing status was independent of marijuana and cigarette use. Also among self-reported alcohol users, housing status was independent of the number of drinks consumed in one setting and self-reported drunkenness. Taken together, these results indicate that there are few behavioral differences that reliably distinguish public housing and conventional housing youth. The next series of analyses extend this inquiry to include measures of psychosocial functioning.

Effect of Housing Status, Ethnic Group and Gender on Alcohol Consumption and Psychosocial Risk

Table 1 contains the results of analyses of variance for the behavioral outcomes and measures of psychosocial functioning. In these analyses, we included race and type (and the interaction of race × type) and, separately, gender and type (and the interaction of gender × type) as independent predictors. The far right-hand column of this table contains the results of tests for significant interactions. Among the alcohol measures, a significant housing status × ethnic group interaction was obtained for perceived alcohol availability, $F(3, 1237) = 3.86$, $p < .05$, with African-American public housing youth ($M = 2.57$) reporting more availability, followed respectively by African-American ($M = 2.54$) and Hispanic youth ($M = 2.54$) living in conventional housing and Hispanic public housing youth ($M = 2.31$). A significant housing status × race interaction was also obtained for drinking intensity, $F(3, 1229) = 6.42$, $p < .01$, with Hispanic housing youth reporting drinking more intensely (more drinks per drinking occasion) compared to African-American housing youth ($Ms = 1.69$ vs. 1.28) and public housing youth drinking more intensely than Hispanic ($M = 1.48$) or African-American ($M = 1.38$) youth living in conventional housing. None of the housing status × gender interactions were significant, although there were several significant main effects for gender (discussed below).

Among the psychosocial measures, there was a significant race × housing status interaction for absenteeism, $F(3, 1248) = 7.91$, $p < .001$, with conventional housing Hispanic youth reporting more absent days compared to conventional housing African-American adolescents ($Ms = 3.33$ vs. 2.69). There was a marginally significant interaction for grades ($p < .10$) and a *post hoc* examination of the means show that Hispanic public housing youth reported lower grades than the remaining three groups. Also, there was a marginal trend for African-American conventional housing youth to report less anxiety and depression than Hispanic conventional housing youths, $F(3, 294) = 3.87$, $p = .05$.

Mean comparisons based on gender for the social influence measures indicated that females reported higher levels of: perceived peer alcohol use, $t(1242) = 6.22$, $p < .0001$; perceived adult alcohol use, $t(1252) = 2.10$, $p < .05$; and greater perceived availability of alcohol, $t(1219) = 2.29$, $p < .05$. Males reported more drinking knowledge, $t(1207) = 2.93$, $p < .01$. Several significant main effects based on gender emerged for psychosocial risk. Females reported they were less influenced by drug promotional advertising, $t(785) = 2.86$, $p < .01$, and their parents had more positive attitudes about drug use, $t(308) = 3.23$, $p < .001$. Females also reported higher levels of self-esteem, $t(349) = 3.07$, $p < .01$; greater ethnic identity, $t(335) = 2.65$, $p < .01$; better grades, $t(1245) = 4.89$, $p < .001$; and better communication skills, $t(658) = 4.20$, $p < .001$. Males, on the other hand, reported more assertive skills, $t(980) = 3.21$, $p < .001$.

TABLE 1. Two-Way ANOVAs of Behavioral and Psychosocial Measures for Housing Type by Ethnicity and Gender

Variables	Total	Public housing			
		Males (n = 262)		Females (n = 362)	
Psychosocial Functioning					
School Bonding	52.39[a]	46.42	(26.13)	54.61	(24.36)
Risk-Taking	48.59	47.63	(21.61)	49.23	(19.41)
Antisocial Behavior	30.41	33.19	(23.20)	28.62	(20.75)
Communication Skills	70.26	67.64	(25.14)	73.23	(21.15)
Cognitive Efficacy	70.48	68.92	(24.32)	71.82	(19.06)
Anxiety and Depression	59.12	62.44	(15.44)	56.92	(15.06)
Behavioral Self-Control	56.45	58.91	(20.00)	55.42	(19.21)
Anxiety Reduction	51.98	50.65	(28.62)	52.39	(25.49)
Assertiveness	80.51	82.53	(16.67)	78.10	(16.84)
Perceived Life Chances	82.55	79.87	(23.22)	85.17	(13.68)
Self-Esteem	76.95	74.03	(28.08)	79.97	(20.29)
Ethnic Identity	72.74	10.31	(28.52)	75.88	(24.72)
Family Management	68.14	67.75	(22.72)	69.54	(18.25)
Social Control					
Absenteeism	2.81	2.82	(1.06)	2.87	(1.07)
Church Attendance	4.94	5.02	(2.57)	4.83	(2.53)
Grades	3.53	3.33	(0.90)	3.62	(0.91)
Alcohol Consumption					
Frequency of Alcohol Use	1.20[b]	1.20	(0.39)	1.23	(0.59)
Drinking Intensity	1.39	1.43	(0.99)	1.37	(0.77)
Drunkenness	1.07	1.06	(0.29)	1.08	(0.54)
Social Influences					
Friends' Usage	1.60	1.56	(0.70)	1.65	(0.79)
Perceived Peer Alcohol Use	2.83	2.06	(0.92)	2.36	(1.00)
Perceived Adult Alcohol Use	3.63	3.47	(1.36)	3.75	(1.17)
Perceived Availability of Alcohol	2.52	2.36	(0.95)	2.60	(0.85)
Parents' Attitude to Substance Use	97.49	95.00	(11.51)	98.79	(4.44)
Friends' Attitude to Alcohol	80.04	80.52	(23.13)	79.98	(23.90)
Alcohol Expectancies	85.60	85.71	(15.47)	85.73	(14.62)
Drinking Knowledge	45.51	46.14	(25.26)	43.61	(23.20)
Drug Resistance Skills	75.67	74.65	(29.16)	76.20	(28.68)

TABLE 1 (continued)

Conventional housing				F values		Interactions	
Males (n = 293)		Females (n = 347)		Ethnicity	Gender	E × Type	G × Type
51.65	(28.89)	54.24	(23.57)	1.17	2.02	0.13	1.21
50.60	(24.11)	47.38	(20.83)	0.92	1.11	1.35	0.45
31.55	(22.59)	29.24	(21.21)	1.16	2.63*	1.82	0.78
68.81	(26.14)	73.73	(21.69)	1.70	6.62***	0.45	1.39
68.30	(25.13)	71.90	(20.25)	0.96	1.59	0.26	0.05
59.05	(15.17)	59.05	(16.76)	1.64	1.51	3.87+	2.44
59.00	(22.02)	54.13	(22.45)	0.60	1.93	1.00	0.15
49.27	(29.16)	54.49	(26.52)	0.36	1.25	0.28	0.72
82.45	(16.89)	79.96	(16.19)	0.78	4.01**	0.31	0.82
80.22	(19.95)	83.23	(16.18)	0.31	1.56	0.83	0.31
70.69	(24.60)	79.72	(17.86)	0.26	3.52*	0.05	0.40
65.46	(28.90)	75.85	(25.79)	0.13	2.83*	0.00	0.64
63.66	(26.56)	69.64	(21.02)	0.32	1.60	0.16	0.97
2.72	(1.14)	2.84	(1.15)	9.97***	1.11	7.91**	0.40
4.97	(2.51)	4.97	(2.43)	0.31	0.36	0.83	0.48
3.45	(0.85)	3.68	(0.85)	3.37*	9.05**	2.78+	0.44
1.21	(0.44)	1.18	(0.37)	1.39	0.53	0.61	0.84
1.39	(0.81)	1.40	(0.84)	10.34***	0.23	6.42**	0.49
1.05	(0.32)	1.06	(0.42)	1.86	0.61	3.76+	0.03
1.59	(0.67)	1.59	(0.68)	1.98	0.97	0.95	1.56
2.12	(0.95)	2.47	(1.01)	0.78	11.85***	0.50	0.23
3.61	(1.30)	3.64	(1.23)	0.00	2.44+	0.01	3.12+
2.50	(0.86)	2.59	(0.87)	3.71*	4.61**	3.86*	2.43
95.14	(13.45)	95.58	(4.83)	0.75	3.51*	2.12	0.05
80.46	(20.53)	79.61	(24.51)	0.88	0.03	2.52	0.00
85.10	(14.34)	85.83	(15.82)	0.35	0.14	0.04	0.16
47.58	(25.16)	41.64	(25.83)	0.27	3.48*	0.01	1.39
74.83	(29.22)	76.55	(27.54)	0.49	0.30	0.14	0.00

[a] Scale scores are prorated for missing items and calibrated to 100-point distributions.
[b] Reported as raw mean (and not percentile indexed) for ease of interpretation.
Sample size varies across variables because of missing data (pairwise deletion). Values in parentheses are standard deviations.

^+p = <.10. $^*p$ < .05. $^{**}p$ < .001. $^{***}p$ < .0001.

Results of the Multiple Regression Analyses

The next series of analyses tested the relative predictive value of each of the risk domains in accounting for alcohol involvement. Despite the cross-sectional nature of these data, we based selection for entry in the equation on theoretical considerations and past empirical findings. At each step, we controlled for housing status (entered first) and followed this in sequential order with forward inclusion of the social control (and demographic variables), social influence, expectancy and knowledge items, and measures of psychosocial functioning. Table 2 contains the results of the regression model with forward inclusion. As depicted, following entry of housing status, the first block included demographic and social control measures (i.e., grades, absenteeism, church attendance, nuclear family status, and gender) and accounted for a significant portion of variation in alcohol use, $F(6, 1265) = 3.67$, $p < .001$. Significant predictors included both grades ($\beta = -.07$, $p < .05$) and absenteeism ($\beta = .09$, $p < .001$). Next, we included the social influence measures which yielded an incremental R^2 of .21, $F(9, 1265) = 99.33$, $p < .0001$. Perceived friend's alcohol use ($\beta = .39$, $p < .001$) and perceived peer use ($\beta = .07$, $p < .05$) accounted for most of the predictive variance. Alcohol expectancies (perceived social

TABLE 2. Results of the Exploratory Multiple Regression[a]

Step for entry of risk domains	b	SE	β	F	Cumulative R^2
1. Social control				3.67**	.02
Grades	−.012	.005	−.07	5.91*	
Absenteeism	.012	.004	.09	9.71*	
2. Social influences				99.33***[c]	.21
Peer alcohol use	.009	.004	.07	5.53*	
Friends' alcohol use	.052	.004	.39	189.92***	
3. Cognitive-Affective				11.01***	.23
Alcohol expectancies	−.001	.000	−.12	20.35***	
4. Psychosocial functioning				1.93*	.33
Housing status[b]	−.047	.015	−.16	9.01*	
Sensation-seeking	.001	.000	.18	7.75*	
Self-esteem	−.001	.000	−.17	5.00*	

[a] Forward entry procedure was used to determine order of risk domain.
[b] Housing status included with Step 1 (social control and demographic measures).
[c] Following Step 1 corresponding F-Test indicates significance of subsequent group (risk domain) controlling for previous step (i.e., incremental F-Test).

*$p < .05$. **$p < .001$. ***$p < .0001$.

outcomes from drinking) and drinking knowledge were entered next and accounted for a significant increment in the overall R^2 of .23, $F(11,1182) =$ 11.01, $p < .0001$. A large share of this variance was attributed to alcohol expectancies ($\beta = -.12, p < .0001$, scaled toward more negative expectancies). At the final step, including all of the remaining psychosocial measures in one block, $F(22, 276) = 1.93, p < .05$, housing status emerged as a significant predictor ($\beta = -.16, p < .01$). Additional significant predictors included in this step included risk-taking ($\beta = .18, p < .01$) and self-esteem ($\beta = -.17, p < .05$). The addition of the psychosocial risk domain netted a change in R^2 of .10.

Moderator Effect of Housing Status on Psychosocial Functioning and Alcohol Use

Based on the previous multiple regression findings, we next tested a buffering or moderator relationship for housing status to determine if specific aspects of psychosocial functioning and alcohol use were conditional on housing status. To test this hypothesis, we used moderated multiple regression techniques (Cohen and Cohen, 1983) regressing alcohol consumption on the psychosocial measures, the moderator (housing status) and an interaction term representing the cross-product of housing and psychosocial functioning. These equations were run separately for each of the psychosocial measures. With the exception of housing status (which was coded dichotomously), all of the predictors were centered (Mean = 0) to reduce collinearity (Dunlap and Kemery, 1987). Table 3 contains the results of these analyses.

There were two significant interaction terms including self-reported grades and perceived availability of alcohol as well as two marginally significant interactions including antisocial behavior and depressive (and anxious) symptomatology ($p < .10$). Figure 1 contains plots of the two equations containing significant interactions. Following conventions proposed by Aiken and West (1991), we plotted the regression equations for the conditional values of housing status. Figure 1 contains plots of the respective regression equations for the significant interactions. These plots are an effective means of portraying the shape or form of the relationship between risk and alcohol consumption for the conditional values (public vs. conventional housing). As depicted in Figure 1a, the relationship between grade point average and alcohol use was relatively flat for public housing youth, however, the regression line for conventional housing youth has a steeper downward slope, indicating a protective effect at higher grades. Turning to Figure 1b, the crossover effect is more dramatic and indicates that at higher levels of perceived alcohol availability, public

TABLE 3. Results of Moderated Multiple Regression Analyses

Risk factor and step	b^1	SE	β	t	$R^{2\dagger}$
Self-reported grades	−.020	.005	−.09	−3.13**	.0067
Housing status	−.010	.009	−.02	−0.88	.0006
A × B	.024	.010	.07	2.42*	.0046
Perceived availability of alcohol	.020	.004	.14	4.86***	.0192
Housing status	−.004	.009	−.01	−0.51	.0003
A × B	−.017	.008	−.06	−2.00*	.0032
Antisocial behavior	.003	.000	.25	9.21***	.0629
Housing status	−.003	.008	−.01	−0.33	.0001
A × B	−.001	.000	−.05	−1.70+	.0021
Depression and anxiety	−.002	.000	−.24	−4.29***	.0594
Housing status	−.010	.018	−.03	−0.55	.0010
A × B	.002	.001	.10	1.72+	.0095

[1] Regression weights for final step inclusive of two main effects and interaction term.
[†] Proportion of variance following first step refers to incremental R^2.

$+p < .10.$ $*p < .05.$ $**p < .01.$ $***p < .001.$

housing youth report lower levels of alcohol consumption than conventional housing youth.

In addition to uncovering a protective or buffering effect for housing status using moderator analyses, we also conducted a series of analyses that reinforce the salience of housing status as a predictor of alcohol consumption. Using backward elimination procedures with all 22 predictors in a single regression model, we obtained a final model accounting for 30% of the variance in alcohol use. Included in this final model were housing status ($\beta = -.16, p < .01$), perceived friends' alcohol use ($\beta = .34, p < .001$), perceived peer use ($\beta = .13, p < .05$), sensation-seeking ($\beta = .17, p < .01$), and self-esteem ($\beta = -.21, p < .001$). Importantly, the reduced model lost only 3% of the overall variance (less than 10%) from the full saturated model with 22 predictors.

DISCUSSION

The current study examined the role of contextual (living conditions) and psychosocial risk factors in the etiology of drug use among inner-city youth. Despite evidence that environmental stressors including poverty and increased crime may heighten vulnerability to drug abuse, few studies

FIGURE 1. Moderator Effect of Housing Status

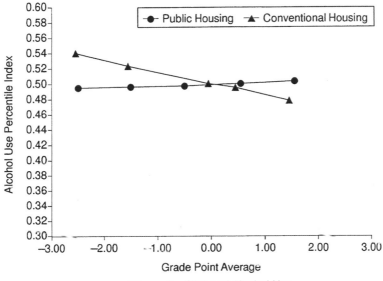

Figure 1a. GPA and Alcohol Use

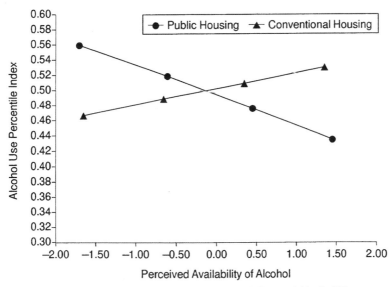

Figure 1b. Perceived Alcohol Availability and Alcohol Use

have examined whether environmental conditions associated with living in public housing developments affect drug abuse risk status. In fact, if poverty and its associated factors is a sufficient condition for drug abuse, then all youth living in impoverished economic conditions would develop drug abuse problems. To address these concerns, we examined the relationship between psychosocial risk and alcohol use among a sample of inner-city public housing youth and a demographically matched comparison group of youth living in conventional housing. By effectively delineating youth residing in housing developments from their surrounding neighborhoods, we sought to determine if contextual features contributed uniquely to the prediction of alcohol use. Housing developments are traditionally located in minority neighborhoods, characterized by high unemployment and high rates of crime (including drug trafficking). Considerable research has shown that continued stressors associated with these conditions may have negative effects on development including poor competence, increased school dropout rates, violence, and inadequate social skills, all of which are antecedent conditions to drug abuse. It is essential, then, to learn if the adaptational skills of these youth are adversely influenced by their exposure to a deleterious environment and whether prevention efforts can focus specifically on building resilience that can retard acquisition of early-stage drug using behaviors.

With regard to consumption, we were unable to distinguish public housing and comparison youth on the basis of self-reported alcohol use. Across both groups, roughly one-third of these youth reported some use of alcohol at an age which is usually associated with initiation to alcohol use (Newcomb and Bentler, 1986). National and regional estimates for the same age group and racial composition indicate similar prevalence estimates, underscoring the similarity of these youth with peers in other regions of the U.S. (Barnes and Welte, 1986; Johnston, O'Malley, and Bachman, 1994). In addition to their similarity on measures of consumption, we were also unable to distinguish the public housing youth and the comparison group on the basis of psychosocial functioning. However, this may not be surprising since the schools these youth attend draw their population from neighborhoods that surround the housing developments from which we drew the housing sample. Therefore, other than the unique conditions associated with the housing development itself, both groups were virtually identical.

There were important findings underscoring the role of ethnicity and gender in promoting alcohol use among inner-city youth. Although we did not find any major pattern that might point toward heightened risk (or protective) status among any particular subgroup, a few trends emerged.

First, females perceived greater alcohol availability than males and this was true for youth living in both types of housing conditions. Within housing developments, African-American youth perceived more alcohol availability than Hispanic youth; however, Hispanic youth reported drinking more intensely (more drinks per drinking occasion) than their African-American counterparts. In terms of psychological functioning, females reported greater self-esteem, more ethnic identity, and better grades than males.

A more complicated picture emerges, however, when we examined interactions between psychosocial functioning, housing status, and alcohol consumption. Superior grades were protective for youth living in conventional housing, lowering their alcohol consumption; whereas grades neither adversely influenced or protected public housing youth. The perception of the availability of alcohol, on the other hand, reduced actual consumption for public housing youth and increased consumption for conventional housing youth. The fact that exposure to peer and/or adult models and the perceived availability of alcohol had a differential impact on alcohol use for public housing and conventional housing youth supports Newcomb and Bentler's (1986) contention of differential exposure and differential vulnerabilities. These authors suggest that, during vicarious learning trials, acquisition of alcohol-related behaviors may result from the extent of exposure and the impact of the model on the observer. Exposure may be heightened or lessened by environmental factors which may affect the number or salience of alcohol-using models, but moderated by protective-enhancing conditions (e.g., strong religious commitment or institutional ties to family). Thus, conditions of vulnerability such as poor academic performance, when combined with environmental stressors, may provide the context for an interactive relationship between exposure and vulnerability. We explored this possibility in the current study and found partial support for conditional effects. In essence, many of these youth come home from school to rundown tenement buildings located in neighborhoods with few parks and recreational activities and, in some cases, to adults who are using drugs. On the other hand, some protective factors may reduce the negative influence produced by these conditions. Moreover, the perception of widespread alcohol use by adults may decrease adolescents' motivations to drink if the adult models are viewed negatively.

This study has several limitations which deserve comment. First, because this study was exploratory, we did not test directional hypotheses and included multiple tests within a single analytic framework increasing the risk of Type I error. Second, housing status was based on self-report data by participating students and was limited to whether they lived in an identified housing development. Future studies should include data from a broad array of variables posited to influence drug use risk as well as the data needed to more precisely classify youth in terms of their housing status.

Another potential limitation is the fact that this study systematically excluded dropout and truant youth, which some have argued represents a loss of individuals who have more serious levels of drug involvement (e.g., Mensch and Kandel, 1988; Kandel, 1975). In particular, the loss of housing development youth who are either truant or highly delinquent and drug-abusing dropouts may conservatively bias our estimates of self-reported drug use. Finally, the cross-sectional nature of these data prevent us from exploring developmental trends that might accentuate drug abuse. For instance, if housing developments are associated with heightened risk it may be that as they get older, housing development youth are forced to choose between remaining in school or dropping out to deal drugs and participate in delinquent activities for economic gain. National educational statistics reveal that between 15 and 18 years of age dropout rates dramatically increase (Statistical Abstracts of the United States, 1995). Our sample was 13-14 years of age, which may prevent us from exploring some of the developmental processes that culminate in delinquent behavior. Future studies are warranted that follow these youth over time in order to track the development of conditions that promote drug abuse.

Current school-based drug abuse prevention programs encompass a broad range of risk reduction strategies aimed at attenuating or eliminating early-stage drug use (Botvin and Botvin, 1992). As such, these programs include a combination of prevention modalities aimed at correcting misperceptions regarding peer and adult drug norms, building self-esteem, imparting social skills (both drug refusal and more general assertiveness skills), and enhancing personal competence (decision-making, self-reinforcement, and self-management skills). Prior research (e.g., Botvin, Baker, Dusenbury, Botvin, and Diaz, 1995; Pentz, Dwyer, MacKinnon, Flay, Hansen, Wang, and Johnson, 1989) provides empirical support for these approaches with a broad range of adolescents. Nonetheless, targeting specific high-risk populations remains an important issue for prevention and has been increasingly regarded as a major component of a more effective national public health agenda.

REFERENCES

Aiken, L. S., & West, S. G. (1991). *Multiple regression: Testing and interpreting interactions*. Newbury Park: Sage Publications.

Barnes, G. M., & Welte, J. W. (1986). Adolescent alcohol abuse: Subgroup differences and relationships to other problem behaviors. *Journal of Adolescent Research, 1*, 79-94.

Baron, R. M., & Kenny, D. A. (1986). The moderator-mediator variable distinction in social psychological research: Conceptual, strategic, and statistical considerations. *Journal of Personality and Social Psychology, 51,* 1173-1182.

Botvin, G. J. (1993). *Reducing drug abuse and AIDS risk: Final Report.* National Institute on Drug Abuse.

Botvin, G. J., Baker, E., Dusenbury, L., Botvin, E., & Diaz, T. (1995). Long-term follow-up of a randomized drug abuse prevention trial in a white middle-class population. *Journal of the American Medical Association, 273,* 1106-1112.

Botvin, G. J., & Botvin, E. M. (1992). *School-based and community-based prevention approaches.* In J. H. Lowinson, P. Ruiz, & R. B. Millman (Eds.), Substance abuse: A comprehensive textbook (2nd ed., pp. 910-927). Baltimore, MD: Williams & Wilkins.

Brook, J. S., Lukoff, I. F., & Whiteman, M. (1977). Peer, family and personality domains as related to adolescents' drug behavior. *Psychological Reports, 41,* 1095-1102.

Brunswick, A. F., & Messeri, P. (1983-84). Causal factors in onset of adolescents' cigarette smoking: A prospective study of urban Black youth. *Advances in Alcohol and Substance Abuse, 3,* 35-52.

Cohen, J., & Cohen, P. (1983). *Applied multiple regression/correlation analysis for the behavioral sciences* (2nd ed.). Hillsdale, NJ: Erlbaum.

Danziger, S. K. (1995). Family life and teenage pregnancy in the inner-city: Experiences of African American youth. *Children & Youth Services Review, 17,* 183-202.

Dembo, R., Allen, N., Farrow, D., Schmeidler, J., & Burgos, W. (1985). A causal analysis of early drug involvement in three inner-city neighborhood settings. *The International Journal of Addictions, 20,* 1213-1237.

Dembo, R., Burgos, W., Des Jarlais, D., & Schmeidler, J. (1979). Ethnicity and drug use among urban junior high school youths. *The International Journal of the Addictions, 14,* 557-568.

Dembo, R., Schmeidler, J., Burgos, W., & Taylor, R. (1985). Environmental setting and early drug involvement among inner-city junior high school youths. *The International Journal of the Addictions, 20,* 1239-1255.

Douglass, F. M., & Khavari, K. A. (1982). A major limitation of the percentile index of overall drug use indulgence. *The International Journal of Addictions, 17,* 283-294.

Dunlap, W. P., & Kemery, E. R. (1987). Failure to detect moderating effects: Is multicollinearity the problem? *Psychological Bulletin, 102,* 418-420.

Durant, R. H., Pendergrast, R. A., & Candenhead, C. (1994). Exposure to violence and victimization and fighting behavior by urban black adolescents. *Journal of Adolescent Health, 15,* 31-38.

Elliot, D. S., Huizinga, D., & Menard, S. (1989). *Multiple problem youth: Delinquency, substance use, and mental health problems.* New York: Springer-Verlag.

Epstein, J. A., Botvin, G. J., Diaz, T., & Schinke, S. P. (1994). The role of social factors and individual characteristics in promoting alcohol among inner-city minority youth. *Journal of Studies on Alcohol, 56,* 39-46.

Farrell, A. D., Danish, S. J., & Howard, C. (1992). Risk factors for drug use in urban adolescents: Identification and cross-validation. *American Journal of Community Psychology, 20,* 263-286.

Figueira-McDonough, J. (1992). Community context and dropout rates. Special issue: Child welfare policy and practice: Rethinking the history of our certainties. *Children and Youth Services Review, 14,* 273-288.

Garmezy, N. (1985). Stress-resistant children: The search for protective factors. In J. E. Stevenson (Ed.), *Recent research in developmental psychopathology* (pp. 213-233). Elmsford, NY: Pergamon Press.

Hawkins, J. D., Catalano, R. F., & Miller, J. L. (1992). Risk and protective factors for alcohol and other drug problems in adolescence and early adulthood: Implications for substance prevention. *Psychological Bulletin, 112,* 351-362.

Johnston, L. D., O'Malley, P. M., & Bachman, J. G. (1994). *National Survey Results on Drug Use from the Monitoring the Future Study, 1975-1993. Vol. I Secondary School Students* (DHHS Publication No. ADM 94-3809). Rockville, MD: National Institute on Drug Abuse.

Kandel, D. (1975). Reaching the hard-to-reach: Illicit drug use among high school absentees. *Addictive Diseases: An International Journal, 1,* 465-480.

Lu, K. H. (1974). The indexing and analysis of drug indulgence. *The International Journal of Addictions, 9,* 785-840.

McLaughlin, M. W., Irby, M. A., & Langman, J. (1994). Urban sanctuaries: Neighborhood organizations in the lives and futures of inner-city youth. San Francisco: Jossey-Bass.

McLoyd, V. C. (1995). Poverty, parenting, and policy: Meeting the support needs of poor parents. In H. E. Fitzgerald, B. M. Lester, & B. S. Zuckerman (Eds.), *Children of poverty: Research, health, and policy issues* (pp. 269-303). New York: Garland Publishing, Inc.

Mensch, B. S., & Kandel, D. B. (1988). Dropping out of high school and drug involvement. *Sociology of Education, 61,* 95-113.

Newcomb, M. D., & Bentler, P. M. (1986). *Consequences of adolescent drug use: Impact on the lives of young adults.* Newbury Park: Sage.

New York City Housing Authority. (1994). *Housing Police Statistics-Incident Report.* New York, NY.

Pentz, M. A., Dwyer, J. H., MacKinnon, D. P., Flay, B. R., Hansen, W. B., Wang, E. Y., & Johnson, C. A. (1989). A multicommunity trial of primary prevention of adolescent drug abuse: Effects on drug use prevalence. *Journal of the American Medical Association, 261,* 3259-3267.

Petraitis, J., Flay, B. R., & Miller, T. Q. (1995). Reviewing theories of adolescent substance use: Organizing pieces in the puzzle. *Psychological Bulletin, 117,* 67-86.

Scheier, L. M., & Botvin, G. J. (1995). *Psychosocial risk factors for adolescents substance use among Hispanic and African American youth: The contributions of ethnicity and ethnic identity.* Unpublished Manuscript. Cornell University Medical College.

Social Indicators. (1995). *The 1995 Annual Report on Social Indicators*. Department of City Planning, City of New York.

Spencer, M. B., Brookins, G. K., & Allen, W. R. (1985). *Beginnings: Social and affective development of Black children*. Hillsdale, NJ: Erlbaum Publishing Company.

Statistical Abstracts of the United States. (1995). *The National Data Book*. U.S. Department of Commerce. Economics and Statistics Administration. Bureau of the Census.

Vergara, C. J. (1989). Hell in a very tall place. *The Atlantic Monthly*, September, pp. 72-78.

Williams, T., & Kornblum, W. (1995). Public housing projects as successful environments for adolescent development. *Annals of the New York Academy of Sciences*, *749*, 153-176.

Factors Associated with Drug Use Among Youth Living in Homeless Shelters

Tracy Diaz
Linda Dusenbury
Gilbert J. Botvin
Rebecca Farmer-Huselid

SUMMARY. There have been only a limited number of studies that examine drug use among homeless youth and there have been no studies to date on drug use with adolescents living in homeless families. This study examined predictors of tobacco, alcohol, and marijuana use with homeless adolescents and preadolescents (N = 234) living in shelters for homeless families. Structured interviews were conducted on self-reported drug use, as well as background variables, social environmental influences, and individual characteristics hypothesized to promote drug use. Logistic-regression analyses revealed that social influences (friends and family drug use) are strong predictors of experimental drug use and intentions to use drugs, as are several psychological factors (psychological well-being, assertiveness, and social support). Implications of the findings for effective prevention programs for homeless and other high risk youth are discussed. *[Article copies available for a fee from The Haworth Document Delivery Service: 1-800-342-9678. E-mail address: getinfo@haworth.com]*

Tracy Diaz, MA, Linda Dusenbury, PhD, and Gilbert J. Botvin, PhD, are affiliated with the Institute for Prevention Research, Cornell University Medical College, 411 East 69th Street, New York, NY 10021. Rebecca Farmer-Huselid is affiliated with Hunter College, City University of New York.

[Haworth co-indexing entry note]: "Factors Associated with Drug Use Among Youth Living in Homeless Shelters." Diaz, Tracy et al. Co-published simultaneously in *Journal of Child & Adolescent Substance Abuse* (The Haworth Press, Inc.) Vol. 6, No. 1, 1997, pp. 91-110; and: *The Etiology and Prevention of Drug Abuse Among Minority Youth* (ed: Gilbert J. Botvin, and Steven Schinke) The Haworth Press, Inc., 1997, pp. 91-110. Single or multiple copies of this article are available for a fee from The Haworth Document Delivery Service [1-800-342-9678, 9:00 a.m. - 5:00 p.m. (EST). E-mail address: getinfo@haworth.com].

KEYWORDS. Drug Use, Homeless, Adolescents

Homelessness is a multi-dimensional phenomenon. More than a lack of housing, homelessness is linked with poverty, abuse, unemployment, and low education (Milburn and D'Ercole, 1991). In and of itself, homelessness can be a major source of life stress. Recent data indicate that an increasing number of families, almost exclusively comprised of women and their children, find themselves in this difficult situation (Milburn and D'Ercole, 1991). Specifically, families comprise more than 30% of the homeless population (U.S. Conference of Mayors, 1987). In New York City, 76% of homeless families are headed by females. In general, the New York City homeless population is becoming increasingly younger (54% of head of households are under 29 years of age) and more in need of social services. Forty-five percent of heads of households did not complete high school, 47% had a child under 2 years old, and 42% indicated serious health, mental health, and/or alcohol/drug problems (NYC Department of Homeless Services, 1993).

Given the multiple stressors faced by homeless families, it is not surprising that homeless children generally show greater dysfunction and lower levels of psychosocial adjustment than housed families. Homeless children are more likely to suffer from health problems, have low school achievement, have more stressful life events, suffer from depression and/or anxiety, have low self-esteem and have other psychosocial problems (Bassuk and Rosenberg, 1990; Bassuk, Rubin, and Lauriat, 1986; Masten, Miliotis, Graham-Bermann, Ramirez, and Neemann, 1993; Rafferty and Shinn, 1991; Wood, Valdez, Hayashi, and Shen, 1990a).

While research on the impact of homelessness on the health and psychological functioning of children is growing, there have been only a limited number of studies that examine drug use among homeless youth. These studies have focused on adolescents who have run away or been forced to leave home. This group of homeless adolescents is typically older and has high rates of problem behaviors, including drug and alcohol abuse, that are often a contributing factor to their homeless status. For example, Greenblatt and Robertson (1993) found 39% of homeless adolescents in Los Angeles met the DSM-III criteria for drug abuse and 48% met it for alcohol dependence. Nine percent of these adolescents indicated that their own drug use was responsible for their being homeless and 46% cited the cause to be other problems, such as arrest or pregnancy. Studies on homeless youth living in homeless families have primarily focused on preschoolers and elementary school-aged children. Adolescents living in homeless families have rarely been studied, and there have been no studies to date on drug use with this population.

The purpose of the current study was to examine a model of potential predictors of drug use and intentions to use drugs for youth living in homeless shelters. Our work was guided by a comprehensive psychosocial framework developed by Jessor (1991) for explaining adolescent risk behavior (problem behavior theory) that includes social environment, perceived environment, and personality factors. Social influences for the individual to use drugs include peers, friends, adults and family members. These influences are included as risk factors in Jessor's problem behavior theory under the rubric of perceived environmental factors.

The importance of social influence factors, including family drug use and family attitudes, low family bonding, peer approval of drug use, associating with drug using peers, and normative expectations of drug use by both adults and peers, for predicting adolescent drug use in white middle-class populations has been well established (Bauman, Botvin, Botvin, and Baker, 1992; Botvin, Botvin, Baker, Dusenbury, and Goldberg, 1992; Fleming, Kellam, and Brown, 1982; Hansen, Graham, Sobel et al., 1987; Hundleby and Mercer, 1987; Jessor and Jessor, 1977; Kandel, 1986; Kandel and Andrew, 1987). Current research has begun to establish the importance of the same social influence factors for predicting drug use among inner-city minority youth (Botvin, Baker, Botvin, Dusenbury, Cardwell, and Diaz, 1993; Botvin, Epstein, Schinke, and Diaz, 1994; Dusenbury, Kerner, Baker, Botvin, James-Ortiz, and Zauber, 1992; Dusenbury, Epstein, Botvin, and Diaz, 1994; Epstein, Botvin, Diaz, Toth, and Schinke, 1995; Epstein, Botvin, Diaz, and Schinke, 1995). Although it is likely that family, peers, and demographic factors predict drug use for all adolescents, it is necessary to confirm that these primary factors are relevant to youth living in homeless shelters, as well as to identify any other pertinent determinants that may be unique to the homeless situation.

The social environment of adolescents living in homeless families differs in several important respects from housed poor adolescents. Homeless adolescents have fewer opportunities for positive adult relations and are more likely to be exposed to drug use in their immediate environment. While homeless mothers have been found to have lower rates of drug use than homeless women without children or homeless mothers who are separated from their children, they have higher rates than housed poor mothers (Bassuk and Rosenberg, 1988; Wood, Valdez, Hayashi, and Shen, 1990b). Homeless children have been found to have less adult support, in general, than housed poor children (Masten et al., 1993). And, while few studies have been done on the relationships between homeless parents and children, Bassuk, Rubin, and Lauriat (1986) report that 25%

of homeless mothers list their children as a primary source of social support.

Homeless children are often isolated from normal peer relations. Homeless families tend to move often (Bassuk and Rosenberg, 1990), consequently homeless youth have a greater number of school changes and are more likely to have friendships disrupted than housed children living in extreme poverty (Masten et al., 1993). Moreover, homeless children face the stigma of homelessness and are more likely to be rejected by their peer group. Children living in temporary housing report feeling ostracized and labeled in their new schools as "shelter kids" (Dusenbury, Botvin, and James-Ortiz, 1989). Masten et al. (1993) found homeless children were less likely to have a close friend or to spend time in the past week with a friend, and twice as many homeless children than housed children reported spending no time at all with a friend in the past week.

Homeless adolescents who spend more time with their friends have to go to great lengths in order to do so. In a study of homeless youth living in temporary housing in New York City, Dusenbury and Diaz (1995) found adolescents reported traveling for up to two hours on weekends to their old neighborhoods to visit their friends, as opposed to making new friends at the shelter. At a time when peer influences are increasing and parent influences decreasing, as the result of normal psychosocial development, homeless adolescents find themselves more isolated from their peers than housed youth. Thus, homeless youth not only experience more environmental stress than housed youth, but also have more limited sources of support from adults and peers.

Risk and protective factors for drug use can be divided into three domains: background variables (age, gender, academic performance); perceptions of the social environmental influences to use drugs (friends' use, friends' attitudes, peer drug norms, adult drug norms); and individual characteristics (self-esteem, risk-taking, assertiveness, support). The purpose of the current study was to examine this comprehensive set of potential predictors of drug use from these domains among homeless youth.

This study examined six measures of drug use: experimental use of cigarettes, alcohol and marijuana, as well as intentions to smoke cigarettes, drink beer or wine, and to use marijuana. A strength of the study is the inclusion of three age groups: preadolescents (9-11), early adolescents (12-14), and middle adolescents (15-16). By using younger adolescents and including measures of intentions, we could examine the factors which promote early experimentation with drugs. This information is important to help identify potentially effective prevention approaches for homeless youth and similar high risk populations.

METHOD

Subjects

Subjects were 234 adolescents and preadolescents living in three Tier II housing shelters in New York City. Subjects were interviewed as part of a larger study on drug abuse prevention with homeless adolescents. The sample was predominately African-American and Hispanic, with 51.1% identifying themselves as African-American, 44% Hispanic, 2.1% white, and 2.8% other. Children's age ranged from 9 to 15 with a mean age of 11.8 years old. The mean grade level was 6th grade. Fifty percent of the children were male. Subjects had spent an average of 6.97 months in the shelter system.

Measures

Children completed face-to-face structured interviews. The interview consisted of 159 items including self-reported drug use and intentions to use drugs in the future, background information, social influence variables, and individual characteristics. The interview took approximately 1 hour and 15 minutes to complete and was conducted in English or in Spanish for those participants who felt more comfortable responding in Spanish.

Background variables. Self-reported data concerning the characteristics of subjects were collected. These included each participant's gender, age, race and academic achievement.

Drug use. Questions about both drug use and drug use intentions were asked for cigarettes, alcohol, and marijuana. For frequency of drug use, children were asked how often they used each substance, with response categories consisting of 1 (never tried it), 2 (tried it but don't use it now), 3 (less than once a month), 4 (about once a month), 5 (about two or three times a month), 6 (about once a week), 7 (a few times a week), 8 (about once a day), and 9 (more than once a day). Three items assessed future use of cigarettes, alcohol, and marijuana within the next year. Participants rated their intention to smoke cigarettes, drink beer or wine, or smoke marijuana during the next year on a five-point scale ranging from 1 (definitely not) to 5 (definitely will).

Social influence variables. A variety of social influences to smoke cigarettes, drink alcoholic beverages, or smoke marijuana were assessed. These include: (1) perceived attitudes of friends toward respondents' use of each substance (friends' attitudes); (2) perceived attitudes of parents toward respondents' use (parents' attitudes); (3) prevalence of use among friends (friends' use); (4) perceived prevalence of use among peers (peer norms); (5) perceived prevalence of use among adults (adult norms); and (6) prevalence of cigarette smoking among family members (mother's smoking, father's smoking, and siblings' smoking). Ratings of friends' attitudes and parents' attitudes were on separate five-point scales ranging from "strongly against it" to "strongly in favor of it." Participants indicated the proportion of their friends, peers, and adults in general who use each drug on separate five-point scales ranging from "none" to "all or almost all." Smoking by older siblings was measured on a five-point scale; responses included "have no older brothers or sisters," "none," "one," "two," and "three or more." Smoking by parents was assessed in separate items for the respondent's father and mother ("Does your father [mother] smoke cigarettes?"). Responses included "have no father/mother," "no," "used to but quit," and "yes."

Individual characteristics. General psychological characteristics or tendencies were also assessed. These included: self-esteem, assertiveness, risk-taking, psychological well-being, the amount of social support received in the past month and satisfaction with that support. An empirically reduced 10-item version of the Rosenberg (1965) scale was used to measure self-esteem (alpha = .89). Responses on the five-point scale ranged from "strongly disagree" to "strongly agree." Statements were typical evocations of self-esteem ("I take a positive attitude toward myself" and "I feel that I have a number of good qualities"). Psychological well-being (alpha = .59) was measured using a 12-item scale (Veit and Ware, 1983). Items concerned self-statements about the frequency of feeling rested, happy, and relaxed in the past month. Responses on the five-point scale ranged from "none of the time" to "most of the time." Students also rated seven items taken from the Eysenck Risk-Taking Scale (Eysenck and Eysenck, 1975) on a five-point scale ranging from "strongly disagree" to "strongly agree" (alpha = .74). The items describe a preference for risk ("I would enjoy fast driving" and "I think life with no danger in it would be dull for me"). Assertiveness was assessed with an abbreviated 18-item version (alpha = .82) of an instrument developed by Gambrill and Richey (Gambrill and Richey, 1975). The items from the Assertion Inventory were rated on five-point scales ranging from "never" to "almost always." Assertiveness was assessed in terms both of resisting drug use offers and general assertiveness. Examples of assertive behavior include returning defective merchandise, complaining when someone steps ahead in line, and saying "no" in various situations. The Arizona Social Support Interview Schedule (Barrera, 1981; Barrera, Sandler, and Ramsay, 1981) was adapted to measure support networks. Participants were asked to name up to four people they would confide in if they needed to talk about something personal and private, and four people they would expect to hear positive feedback from. They were also asked to indicate whether or not they received the support in the past month. An additional measure of support was included to assess the amount of satisfaction the individual felt with the level of support received. For support from confidants, subjects were asked if in the past month they would have liked (1) "a lot more opportunities to talk to people about personal and private feelings," (2) "a few more opportunities," or (3) "was this about right." For support from positive feedback, subjects were asked if they would have liked people to have told them they liked their ideas or liked the things they did (1) "a lot more," (2) "a little more," or (3) "was it about right."

Procedure

Participants were recruited by utilizing flyers distributed throughout the shelter, shelter staff (individual caseworkers), word-of-mouth, and telephone solicitations made by interviewers. As part of the larger study, an entire family (one parent and all eligible children) were asked to participate. Only children between the ages of 9 to 15 were eligible for the interview. Interviews were conducted outside of the family's room, in a public common room. Parents and children were either interviewed at separate times or in separate rooms, so children would feel comfortable answering honestly. Incentives were offered for completing the interview. Mothers were paid $15 for their interview and $5 for each of their children who completed an interview. Incentives were only paid after the entire family had completed the interview. Data were collected on an ongoing basis at each shelter for a period of six months.

Data Analysis

Correlations were computed to determine the relationship between each of the drug use measures and the background variables, the social influence variables, and the individual characteristics. A series of logistic regression analyses were conducted to determine which of the variables associated with drug use were the most important predictors of drug use for homeless youth. Drinking and marijuana use indexes were collapsed into two categories: ever used (alcohol, 72%; marijuana, 92%) versus never used (alcohol, 28%; marijuana, 8%). Due to a small number of smokers in the sample, a logistic regression model was not run on experimental smoking. Behavioral intention measures were collapsed into two categories: intention to definitely not use (cigarettes, 78%; beer or wine, 79%; marijuana, 93%) versus intention to use or undecided about using in the future (cigarettes, 22%; beer or wine, 21%; marijuana, 7%). For each dependent variable, three logistic regressions were computed, one for each of the three variable domains in the study (background variables, social influence variables, and individual characteristics). Significant predictors from each of the three logistic regressions were included in the final logistic regression models for each dependent variable. Individuals for whom any of the variables in the equation were missing were omitted from the analysis.

RESULTS

Drug Use and Predictor Variables

Table 1 reports the relationship between each measure of drug use (smoking, drinking, and marijuana use) and the predictor variables. For the background variables, both age and academic achievement significantly correlated with each measure of drug use. Gender and race, however, were unrelated to any measure of drug use.

In the social influence domain, friends' attitudes toward the use of each drug and friends' use of each drug were significantly correlated with all drug indexes. Peer norms were related to drinking and marijuana use, but not to smoking. Adult norms were significantly correlated only with drinking, and parent attitudes were related only to smoking. Mothers' smoking was related to drinking frequency only, fathers' smoking was related to smoking only, and siblings' smoking was related to both smoking and marijuana use. No relationships were observed between individual characteristics and drug use.

Drug Use Intentions and Predictor Variables

Table 2 reports the relationship between predictor variables and intentions to smoke cigarettes, drink beer or wine, and use marijuana in the next year. Significant correlations between age and academic achievement and intentions to drink and to use marijuana were found, but not for intentions to smoke cigarettes. No relationships were found between gender or race and any of the drug use intention variables.

In the social influence domain, friends' attitudes and friends' use of drugs were again significantly correlated with the adolescent's intentions to use each substance. Peer norms were also correlated with both intentions to drink beer or wine and intentions to use marijuana, and adult

TABLE 1. Correlations Between Drug Use Variables and Predictor Variables

	Smoking Index	Drinking Index	Marijuana Index
Background			
Age	.27***	.36***	.26***
Academic Achievement	.24***	.32***	.23**
Sex	.04	.05	.08
Race	−.02	.12	−.02
Social Influence			
Adult Norms	.05	.19**	.12
Peer Norms	.12	.29***	.21**
Parent Attitudes	.37***	.11	.10
Friends' Attitudes	.26***	.32***	.40***
Friends' Use	.32***	.55***	.61***
Mother Smoking	.06	.18**	−.02
Father Smoking	.13*	.02	−.03
Sibling Smoking	.26***	.07	.22**
Individual			
Self-Esteem	.01	.06	−.01
Risk-Taking	.02	.05	.10
Assertiveness	−.04	.02	−.04
Wellness	.02	−.03	−.02
Confidant Support	.02	.03	.10
Feedback Support	−.05	.10	.00
Confidant Satisfaction	.06	−.07	.08
Feedback Satisfaction	.03	.02	.07

*$p < .05$, **$p < .01$, ***$p < .001$

norms were significantly correlated with only intentions to drink beer or wine. Parents' attitudes were significantly related to adolescent intentions to drink beer or wine, but not related to intentions to smoke cigarettes or use marijuana. Mothers' smoking was also related to intention to drink beer or wine. Fathers' smoking had no relationship to drug use intentions and siblings' smoking was only related to intentions to smoke marijuana.

For individual characteristics, assertiveness was negatively related to intentions to smoke and not at all related to intentions to drink beer or wine or to use marijuana. Psychological well-being was negatively related to intentions to drink beer or wine and had no relationship with intentions to smoke or use marijuana. Amount of positive feedback received was negatively related to intentions to use cigarettes, but not related to either intentions to drink beer or wine or to use marijuana. No other individual characteristic was related to the drug use intention variables.

TABLE 2. Correlations Between Drug Use Intentions and Predictor Variables

	Intention to Smoke Cigarettes	Intention to Drink Beer or Wine	Intention to Use Marijuana
Background			
Age	.12	.28***	.26***
Academic Achievement	.08	.24***	.20**
Sex	−.06	.08	−.02
Race	−.02	−.02	−.04
Social Influence			
Adult Norms	.05	.20**	.12
Peer Norms	.08	.28***	.27***
Parent Attitudes	.10	.30***	.08
Friends' Attitudes	.19**	.24***	.44***
Friends' Use	.30***	.38***	.58***
Mother Smoking	.05	.19**	.07
Father Smoking	−.03	.02	−.00
Sibling Smoking	.10	.09	.15*
Individual			
Self-Esteem	.07	.05	−.03
Risk-Taking	.10	.06	−.06
Assertiveness	−.18**	.00	−.11
Wellness	−.13	−.16*	−.00
Confidant Support	−.07	−.08	.03
Feedback Support	−.18**	−.01	−.03
Confidant Satisfaction	.01	−.05	.08
Feedback Satisfaction	.09	.11	.10

*$p < .05$, **$p < .01$, ***$p < .001$

Concurrent Predictors of Drug Use

Tables 3a, b, c show the significant predictors of alcohol and marijuana use. Significant predictors for drinking included friends' use of beer or wine and mothers' smoking status. The odds of trying alcohol were 3.98 times higher for individuals who reported that less than half of their friends drink beer or wine and 17.72 times higher for individuals who reported that 50%-100% of their friends drink beer or wine, compared to individuals who reported that none of their friends drink beer or wine. Individuals who reported that their mother was a current smoker were 3.83 times more likely to drink beer or wine than individuals who reported their mothers did not smoke.

TABLE 3a. Predictors of Cigarette Smoking (Ever Use): Final Logistic Regression Models

Variable	Odds Ratio	95% Confidence Interval	
		Low	High
Age (Preadolescence[a])			
Early Adolescence	4.09	2.19	7.65
Middle Adolescence	3.46	1.49	8.01
Mother Smokes (No[a])			
Yes	1.37	.68	2.78
Wellness (High[a])			
Low	.50	.28	.89

[a]Reference group.

TABLE 3b. Predictors of Drinking (Ever Use): Final Logistic Regression Models

Variable	Odds Ratio	95% Confidence Interval	
		Low	High
Age (Preadolescence[a])			
Early Adolescence	1.44	.62	3.35
Middle Adolescence	1.63	.53	4.99
Friends' Use (None[a])			
Less than 50%	3.98	1.81	8.72
50-100%	17.72	5.13	61.20
Mother Smokes (No[a])			
Yes	3.83	1.30	11.25
Perceived Teen Norms: Beer (Less than Half[a])			
50%	1.70	.68	4.22
50-100%	1.86	.75	4.59
Feedback Support (None[a])			
2 Instances	1.66	.62	4.45
3 or More Instances	1.66	.70	3.93
Wellness (High[a])			
Low	1.73	.84	3.56

[a]Reference group.

TABLE 3c. Predictors of Marijuana Use (Ever Use): Final Logistic Regression Models

Variable	Odds Ratio	95% Confidence Interval	
		Low	High
Age (Preadolescence[a])			
Early Adolescence	1.46	.22	9.72
Middle Adolescence	2.90	.37	22.41
Academic Achievement (High[a])			
Medium	2.82	.62	12.77
Low	6.95	1.18	40.89
Friends' Use (None[a])			
Less than 50%	5.09	1.09	23.70
50-100%	15.11	2.90	78.78
Sibling(s) Smokes (No[a])			
1 or More Sibling Smokes	3.43	1.07	10.98
Wellness (High[a])			
Low	3.80	1.07	13.56

[a]Reference group.

Significant predictors for trying marijuana included academic achievement, friends' use of marijuana, sibling smoking status, and psychological well-being. Individuals with low academic achievement were 6.95 times more likely to have tried marijuana than individuals with high academic achievement. The odds of trying marijuana were 5.09 times higher for individuals who reported that less than 50% of their friends use marijuana and 15.11 times higher for individuals who reported that 50%-100% of their friends use marijuana, compared to individuals who reported that none of their friends use marijuana. Individuals who reported that one or more of their older siblings smoked were 3.43 times more likely to use marijuana than individuals with no older siblings who smoke. Scoring low on the psychological well-being scale increased the odds for trying marijuana 3.80 times.

Concurrent Predictors of Drug Use Intentions

Tables 4a, b, c show the final regression models for each measure of drug use intentions. Intentions to smoke cigarettes were predicted by friends' smoking, amount of positive feedback received, assertiveness, and psycho-

TABLE 4a. Predictors of Intentions to Smoke Cigarettes: Final Logistic Regression Models

		95% Confidence Interval	
Variable	Odds Ratio	Low	High
Friends' Use (None[a])			
Less than 50%	3.14	1.40	7.04
50-100%	4.71	1.80	12.31
Feedback Support (None[a])			
2 Instances	.37	.14	.99
3 or More Instances	.43	.20	.95
Assertiveness (High[a])			
Low	2.56	1.24	5.31
Wellness (High[a])			
Low	2.27	1.11	4.64

[a]Reference group.

logical well-being. The odds of intending to smoke cigarettes were 3.14 times higher for individuals who reported that less than half of their friends smoke cigarettes and 4.71 times higher for individuals who reported that 50%-100% of their friends smoke cigarettes, compared to individuals who reported that none of their friends smoke cigarettes. Individuals who reported two instances of feedback support in the past month were .37 times less likely to intend to smoke cigarettes and individuals who reported three instances of feedback support in the past month were .43 times less likely to intend to smoke cigarettes than individuals who reported no feedback support. The odds of intending to smoke cigarettes were 2.27 times higher for individuals who scored low on the psychological well-being scale and 2.56 times higher for individuals who scored low on the assertiveness scale.

Significant predictors of intentions to drink beer or wine include friends' use of beer or wine, mothers' smoking status, and psychological well-being. The odds of intending to drink beer or wine were 6.60 times higher for individuals who reported that less than half of their friends drink beer or wine and 7.96 times higher for individuals who reported that 50%-100% of their friends drink beer or wine, compared to individuals who reported that none of their friends drink beer or wine. Individuals who reported that their mother currently smokes cigarettes were 4.45 times more likely to intend to drink, compared to individuals who reported their mothers never

TABLE 4b. Predictors of Intentions to Drink: Final Logistic Regression Models

		95% Confidence Interval	
Variable	Odds Ratio	Low	High
Age (Preadolescence[a])			
Early Adolescence	1.61	.57	4.59
Middle Adolescence	3.56	.98	12.98
Academic Achievement (High[a])			
Low	.77	.19	3.14
Medium	2.34	.92	5.94
Mother Smokes (No[a])			
Yes	4.45	1.22	16.26
Friends' Use (None[a])			
Less than 50%	6.60	2.60	16.79
50-100%	7.96	2.37	26.80
Perceived Teen Norms: Beer (Less than Half[a])			
50%	1.00	.33	3.02
50-100%	1.75	.63	4.86
Confidant Support (None[a])			
One Confidant	1.51	.57	4.00
Two Confidants	.93	.26	3.37
Three or More Confidants	.47	.12	1.79
Wellness (High[a])			
Low	2.64	1.14	6.12

[a]Reference group.

smoked. The odds of intending to drink beer or wine were 2.64 times higher for individuals who scored low on the psychological well-being scale.

Significant predictors of intentions to smoke marijuana included expectations of peer marijuana use, assertiveness, and psychological well-being. Individuals who believed that over half of all teenagers smoke marijuana were 11.33 times more likely to intend to try marijuana themselves. The odds of intending to smoke marijuana were 11.21 times higher for individuals who scored low on the psychological well-being scale and 11.19 times higher for individuals who scored low on the assertiveness scale.

TABLE 4c. Predictors of Intentions to Use Marijuana: Final Logistic Regression Models

Variable	Odds Ratio	95% Confidence Interval	
		Low	High
Age (Preadolescence[a])			
Early Adolescence	3.02	.45	20.12
Middle Adolescence	8.77	.84	91.80
Perceived Teen Norms: Marijuana (Less than 50%[a])			
50%	1.16	.16	8.33
50-100%	11.33	1.64	78.28
Confidant Satisfaction (About Right[a])			
A Few More	.16	.01	1.83
A Lot More	.14	.01	1.46
Feedback Satisfaction (About Right[a])			
A Few More	.17	.02	1.79
A Lot More	.27	.04	1.62
Confidant Support (None[a])			
One Confidant	4.33	.62	30.42
Two Confidants	.70	.04	11.50
Three or More Confidants	2.77	.28	27.39
Assertiveness (High[a])			
Low	11.19	2.06	60.81
Wellness (High[a])			
Low	11.21	2.03	61.82

[a]Reference group.

DISCUSSION

This study was designed to increase our understanding of the factors associated with drug use in an understudied population, homeless youth. The factors related to drug use included: age, academic achievement, several social influence variables (friends' use, family's use, and expectations of peer use) as well as various individual characteristics (psychological well-being, assertiveness, and social support).

The only background variable with any predictive power was academic achievement. While this finding is supported by previous research (Bachman, Johnston, and O'Malley, 1981; Fleming, Kellam, and Brown, 1982), academic achievement was not predictive of all drug use outcomes as might be expected, but rather only with marijuana use.

Of the social influence variables, friends' use was the most consistent predictor of drug use for homeless youth. Specifically, the prevalence of drug use among friends predicted drinking and marijuana use as well as intentions to smoke and drink. Furthermore, for homeless youth who believed that more than 50% of teenagers use marijuana, the odds of intending to try marijuana in the next year was more than 11 times greater. These findings replicate those found in previous studies with housed poor adolescents (Botvin et al., 1993; Botvin et al., 1994; Dusenbury et al., 1992; Dusenbury et al., 1994; Epstein, Botvin, Diaz, Toth, and Schinke, 1995). Family smoking status also predicted drug use for homeless youth, although not as consistently as has been found in previous studies. Having a mother who smokes increased the odds of both drinking and intending to drink, but not of intending to smoke. In addition, having at least one older sibling who smokes increased the odds of using marijuana.

Other social influence variables, such as attitudes of both friends and parents towards drug use and perceived adult drug use norms, did not predict drug use in this population. As with both housed poor minority adolescents and with white suburban adolescents, social influences play a critical role in both the initiation of drug use and the intention to use drugs for homeless youth. However, for homeless adolescents it appears that experiencing drug use in their immediate environment (especially through friends' use) is more important in determining their drug use than the attitudes of their families and friends towards drugs or than their general perceptions of drug use in their environment.

With respect to individual characteristics, psychological well-being was the most consistent predictor of drug use. Having low levels of psychological well-being in the past month increased the odds of using marijuana, as well as intending to use all three drugs in the coming year. One explanation for this finding is that the level of distress homeless youth have experienced may promote drug use as a form of self-medication. This is partially supported by the finding that as the amount of social support received in the last month increased, the odds of intending to smoke cigarettes decreased. Although the cross-sectional nature of this study precludes drawing conclusions about the direction of causation, this finding suggests the importance of providing homeless youth with skills for coping with stress as well as increasing the amount of social support.

Another important finding was the predictive power of assertiveness for homeless youths' intentions to smoke cigarettes and to use marijuana.

Being low in assertive skills may increase susceptibility to persuasion and social influences to use drugs. The finding that low assertiveness predicts drug use intentions suggests the need to include general assertive skills, as well as drug resistance skills, in programs designed to prevent the initiation of drug use.

While social influence factors were predictive of drug use among homeless youth, this study did not fully replicate the impact of social influences on adolescent drug use that has been found with other adolescents. It may be that not enough is known about homeless families in general, to understand the lack of social influences on homeless youth's drug use. Homeless families may have undergone separation (i.e., foster-care) over the course of the adolescent's life that have diluted the effect of any family member's own drug use on their child. Homeless families often become homeless after living with extended family members and/or friends in overcrowded conditions (Bassuk and Rosenberg, 1988; Shinn, Knickman, and Weitzman, 1991). It is possible that the social influences in these living situations play a role in predicting drug use among homeless adolescents. It is important to remember in both conducting research and in designing intervention strategies for homeless youth, that homelessness is an event occurring in a developmental continuum. In addition to specific influences and consequences (i.e., isolation from peers and stigmatization) which can result from becoming homeless, it can also be an indicator of a history of poverty, family disruption and instability; all of which may influence drug use outcomes. Additional research should be conducted to better understand the environment of homeless children both prior to and after the event of homelessness.

Results of this study have several implications for developing prevention programs for homeless youth. Prevention approaches designed for homeless youth should (1) provide an awareness of the various social influences to use drugs, (2) incorporate a broad-based social competency approach which teaches drug-refusal skills, general assertiveness skills, stress/anxiety management techniques, and general social skills, and (3) provide opportunities for gaining peer support by building positive peer groups.

Recognizing the inherent limitation of cross-sectional data, it is important to view these findings as suggestive rather than conclusive. Additional research is clearly necessary to determine the extent to which the predictors identified in this study can be replicated with a longitudinal study. Still, this study provides important new data about the etiology of drug use in homeless youth and implications for prevention.

REFERENCES

Bachman, J. G., Johnston, L. K., & O'Malley, P. M. (1981). Smoking, drinking, and drug use among American high school students: Correlates and trends, 1975-1979. *American Journal of Public Health, 71*, 59-69.

Barrera, M. (1981). Social support in the adjustment of pregnant adolescents: Assessment issues. In B. Gottlieb (Ed.), *Social Networks and Social Support* (67-96). Beverly Hills, CA: Sage.

Barrera, M., Sandler, I. N., & Ramsay, T. B. (1981). Preliminary development of a scale of social support: Studies on college students. *American Journal of Community Psychology, 9*, 435-447.

Bassuk, E. L. & Rosenberg, L. (1988). Why does family homelessness occur? A case-control study. *American Journal of Public Health, 78*(7), 783-787.

Bassuk, E. L. & Rosenberg, L. (1990). Psychosocial characteristics of homeless children and children with homes. *Pediatrics, 85*(3), 257-261.

Bassuk, E. L., Rubin, L., & Lauriat, A. S. (1986). Characteristics of sheltered homeless families. *American Journal of Public Health, 76*(9), 1097-1101.

Bauman, K. E., Botvin, G. J., Botvin, E. M., & Baker, E. (1992). Normative expectations and the behavior of significant others: An integration of traditions in research on adolescents' cigarette smoking. *Psychological Reports, 71*, 568-570.

Botvin, G. J., Baker, E., Botvin, E. M., Dusenbury, L., Cardwell, J., & Diaz, T. (1993). Factors promoting cigarette smoking among black youth: A causal modeling approach. *Addictive Behaviors, 18*, 397-405.

Botvin, G. J., Botvin, E. M., Baker, E., Dusenbury, L., & Goldberg, C. J. (1992). The false consensus effect: Predicting adolescents' tobacco use from normative expectations. *Psychological Reports, 70*, 171-178.

Botvin, G. J., Epstein, J. A., Schinke, S., & Diaz, T. (1994). Predictors of cigarette smoking among inner-city minority youth. *Developmental and Behavioral Pediatrics, 15*(2), 67-73.

Dusenbury, L., Botvin, G. J., & James-Ortiz, S. (1989). The primary prevention of adolescent substance abuse through the promotion of personal and social competence. *Prevention in Human Services, 7*, 201-224.

Dusenbury, L. & Diaz, T. (1995). Developing interventions for multiethnic populations: A case study with homeless youth. In G. J. Botvin, S. Schinke, & M. Orlandi (Eds.), *Drug Abuse Prevention with Multiethnic Youth* (169-192). Newbury Park, CA: Sage Publications.

Dusenbury, L., Epstein, J. A., Botvin, G. J., & Diaz, T. (1994). Social influence predictors of alcohol use among New York Latino youth. *Addictive Behaviors, 19*(4), 363-372.

Dusenbury, L., Kerner, J. F., Baker, E., Botvin, G. J., James-Ortiz, S., & Zauber, A. (1992). Predictors of smoking prevalence among New York Latino youth. *American Journal of Public Health, 82*(1), 55-58.

Epstein, J. A., Botvin, G. J., Diaz, T., & Schinke, S. (1995). The role of social factors and individual characteristics in promoting alcohol use among inner-city minority youths. *Journal of Studies on Alcohol, 56,* 39-46.

Epstein, J. A., Botvin, G. J., Diaz, T., Toth, V., & Schinke, S. (1995). Social and personal factors in marijuana use and intentions to use drugs among inner city minority youth. *Developmental and Behavioral Pediatrics, 16*(1), 14-20.

Eysenck, H. J. & Eysenck, S. G. G. (1975). *Manual of the Eysenck Personality Questionnaire.* London: Hodder & Stoughton.

Fleming, J. P., Kellam, S. G., & Brown, C. H. (1982). Early predictors of age at first use of alcohol, marijuana and cigarettes. *Drug and Alcohol Dependency, 9,* 285-303.

Gambrill, E. D. & Richey, C. A. (1975). An assertion inventory for use in assessment and research. *Behavioral Therapy, 6,* 550-561.

Greenblatt, M. & Robertson, M. J. (1993). Life-styles, adaptive strategies, and sexual behaviors of homeless adolescents. *Hospital and Community Psychiatry, 44*(12), 1177-1180.

Hansen, W. B., Graham, J. W., Sobel, J. L., Shelton, D. R., Flay, B. R., & Johnson, C. A. (1987). The consistency of peer and parent influences on tobacco, alcohol, and marijuana use among young adults. *Journal of Behavioral Medicine, 10*(6), 559-579.

Hundleby, J. D. & Mercer, G. W. (1987). Family and friends as social environments and their relationship to young adolescents' use of alcohol, tobacco, and marijuana. *Journal of Clinical Psychology, 44,* 125-134.

Jessor, R. (1991). Risk behavior in adolescence: A psychosocial framework for understanding and action. *Journal of Adolescent Health, 12,* 597-605.

Jessor, R. & Jessor, S. L. (1977). *Problem Behavior and Psychosocial Development: A Longitudinal Study of Youth.* San Diego, CA: Academic Press, Inc.

Kandel, D. B. (1986). Processes of peer influence in adolescence. In R. Silberstein, (Ed.), *Development as Action in Context: Problem Behavior and Normal Youth Development* (203-228). New York: Springer-Verlag.

Kandel, D. B., & Andrew, K. (1987). Processes of adolescent socialization by parents and peers. *International Journal of the Addictions, 22,* 319-342.

Masten, A. S., Miliotis, D., Graham-Bermann, S. A., Ramirez, M., & Neemann, J. (1993). Children in homeless families: Risks to mental health and development. *Journal of Consulting and Clinical Psychology, 61*(2), 335-343.

Milburn, N. & D'Ercole, A. (1991). Homeless women: Moving toward a comprehensive model. *American Psychologist, 46*(11), 1161-1169.

New York City Department of Homeless Services. (1993). New York City Revised and Updated Plan for Housing and Assisting Homeless Single Adults and Families, March 1993.

Rafferty, Y. & Shinn, M. (1991). The impact of homelessness on children. *American Psychologist, 46* (11), 1170-1179.

Rosenberg, M. (1965). *Society and the adolescent self-image.* Princeton: Princeton University Press.

Shinn, M., Knickman, J. R., & Weitzman, B. C. (1991). Relationships and vulnerability to becoming homeless among poor families. *American Psychologist, 46*(11), 1180-1187.

U.S. Conference of Mayors (1987). *The continued growth of hunger, homelessness and poverty in America's cities in 1986.* Washington, DC: Author.

Veit, C. T. & Ware, J. E., Jr. (1983). The structure of psychological distress and well being in general populations. *Journal of Consulting and Clinical Psychology, 51*, 730-742.

Wood, D. L., Valdez, R. B., Hayashi, T., & Shen, A. (1990a). Health of homeless children and housed poor children. *Pediatrics, 86*(6), 858-866.

Wood, D. L., Valdez, R. B., Hayashi, T., & Shen, A. (1990b). Homeless and housed families in Los Angeles: A study comparing demographic, economic, and family function characteristics. *American Journal of Public Health, 80*(9), 1049-1052.

Index

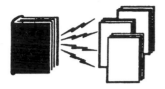

Haworth
DOCUMENT DELIVERY
SERVICE

This valuable service provides a single-article order form for any article from a Haworth journal.

- *Time Saving:* No running around from library to library to find a specific article.
- *Cost Effective:* All costs are kept down to a minimum.
- *Fast Delivery:* Choose from several options, including same-day FAX.
- *No Copyright Hassles:* You will be supplied by the original publisher.
- *Easy Payment:* Choose from several easy payment methods.

Open Accounts Welcome for . . .
- Library Interlibrary Loan Departments
- Library Network/Consortia Wishing to Provide Single-Article Services
- Indexing/Abstracting Services with Single Article Provision Services
- Document Provision Brokers and Freelance Information Service Providers

---

MAIL or *FAX* THIS ENTIRE ORDER FORM TO:

Haworth Document Delivery Service
The Haworth Press, Inc.
10 Alice Street
Binghamton, NY 13904-1580

or FAX: 1-800-895-0582
or CALL: 1-800-342-9678
9am-5pm EST

PLEASE SEND ME PHOTOCOPIES OF THE FOLLOWING SINGLE ARTICLES:
1) Journal Title: _____
   Vol/Issue/Year:_____Starting & Ending Pages:_____
   Article Title:_____
   _____

2) Journal Title: _____
   Vol/Issue/Year:_____Starting & Ending Pages:_____
   Article Title:_____
   _____

3) Journal Title: _____
   Vol/Issue/Year:_____Starting & Ending Pages:_____
   Article Title:_____
   _____

4) Journal Title: _____
   Vol/Issue/Year:_____Starting & Ending Pages:_____
   Article Title:_____
   _____

(See other side for Costs and Payment Information)

COSTS: Please figure your cost to order quality copies of an article.

1. Set-up charge per article: $8.00
   ($8.00 × number of separate articles) _____

2. Photocopying charge for each article:

   1-10 pages: $1.00 _____

   11-19 pages: $3.00 _____

   20-29 pages: $5.00 _____

   30+ pages: $2.00/10 pages _____

3. Flexicover (optional): $2.00/article _____

4. Postage & Handling: US: $1.00 for the first article/
   $.50 each additional article _____

   Federal Express: $25.00 _____

   Outside US: $2.00 for first article/
   $.50 each additional article_____

5. Same-day FAX service: $.35 per page _____

   GRAND TOTAL: _____

METHOD OF PAYMENT: (please check one)

❑ Check enclosed   ❑ Please ship and bill. PO # _____
(sorry we can ship and bill to bookstores only! All others must pre-pay)

❑ Charge to my credit card: ❑ Visa;   ❑ MasterCard;   ❑ Discover;
   ❑ American Express;

Account Number:_____ Expiration date:_____

Signature: *X*_____

Name: _____ Institution: _____

Address: _____

_____

City: _____ State:_____ Zip:_____

Phone Number: _____ FAX Number: _____

MAIL or *FAX* THIS ENTIRE ORDER FORM TO:

Haworth Document Delivery Service
The Haworth Press, Inc.
10 Alice Street
Binghamton, NY 13904-1580

or FAX: 1-800-895-0582
or CALL: 1-800-342-9678
9am-5pm EST)